A HEALTHIER FUTURE?

Managing healthcare in Ireland

Edited by Eilish Mc Auliffe and Laraine Joyce

First published in 1998
by the Institute of Public Administration
57-61 Lansdowne Road
Dublin 4
Ireland

www.ipa.ie

Reprinted 1999

British Library Cataloguing in Publication Data
A catalogue record for this book is available from the British Library.

ISBN 1 902448 02 2

Cover design by Butler Claffey Design, Dun Laoghaire
Typeset by Wendy Commins, The Curragh, Co. Kildare
Printed by Johnswood Press, Dublin

Contents

Contributors

EILISH MC AULIFFE is Director of the MSc in Health Services Management at Trinity College Dublin, and also works with the Midland Health Board as an organisational development specialist. Previously she worked in the Health Services Development Unit at the Institute of Public Administration.

LARAINE JOYCE is Deputy Director of the Office for Health Management. She was formerly an Executive Director of the Institute of Public Administration, with responsibility for its services to the health sector.

PATRICK DOORLEY is Director of Public Health in the Midland Health Board, and a member and fellow of the Faculty of Public Health Medicine of Ireland. He lectures and has published on the subjects of health gain and health and lifestyle.

DAVID McKEVITT is Senior Lecturer in Management and Marketing at the University of Limerick, and has worked in both the public and private sectors. He has been associated with the Department of Finance, University College Cork, and the Open University.

SEAN CONROY is Programme Manager, General Hospital Care, Western Health Board. Dr Conroy worked as an oil exploration engineer and later took up medicine, qualifying in 1983.

MIRIAM HEDERMAN O'BRIEN has chaired the Commission on Health Funding (1987–1989), the Expert Committee Inquiring into the National Blood Transfusion Service Products (1994–1995) and the Independent Review Group, Drogheda (1996). Dr Hederman O'Brien is currently Chancellor of the University of Limerick.

FERGAL LYNCH is an Assistant Principal in the Department of Health. He lectures in Economics, Health Economics and Health Planning at the Institute of Public Administration, and in a number of courses at Masters level.

MARIE BRADY is a Senior Training Specialist in the Health Services Training Unit of the Institute of Public Administration, which she joined in 1986. Previously she worked for a number of years as an economic analyst in the civil service.

PETER WEST has taught at several third-level institutions in Britain, including the London School of Economics, the University of Sussex and the University of Bath, and was a fellow of the King's Fund College. Dr West is currently a Senior Lecturer at the United Medical and Dental Schools of Guy's and St Thomas's Hospitals, London.

DENIS DOHERTY is Chief Executive of the Midland Health Board and Director of the Office for Health Management. He is President of the Standing Committee of the Hospitals of the European Union (HOPE) and a member of the Commission on Nursing and Comhairle na n-Ospidéal.

MAUREEN P. LYNOTT is Director of Provider Affairs with BUPA Ireland. She lectures in Management at Trinity College Dublin, University College Dublin and Dublin City University.

AUSTIN L. LEAHY is a Lecturer in the Department of Surgery at the Royal College of Surgeons in Ireland, and a Consultant Surgeon in Beaumont Hospital. He is Director of the Diploma in Management in the Centre for Healthcare at the Royal College of Surgeons in Ireland, and President of the Irish Society for Quality in Healthcare.

PATRICIA BROWN was Senior Social Research Officer at the Institute of Public Administration, and previously lectured on social policy in the Institute's degree programmes. She currently lectures in the Institute's postgraduate programmes.

TIM O'SULLIVAN is a Health Services Specialist with the Institute of Public Administration, and Co-ordinator of its MA in Healthcare Management. He previously edited *Health Services News*, an annual series of health factsheets and other IPA publications for the health services.

DAVID KENEFICK is Divisional Manager of Clinic Services in St Michael's House's services for people with learning disabilities. He worked at the Institute of Public Administration between 1995 and 1998, first as a full-time Healthcare Management Specialist and then as an Associate Specialist.

GERALDINE McCARTHY is Director of the Department of Nursing Studies, University College Cork. Dr McCarthy has held nursing positions in the UK, the USA, Ireland and Canada.

JOHN KEVANY is a public health physician with extensive experience of primary healthcare systems in the developing world. He has recently been involved in applying the principles of primary healthcare development to special groups and situations in Ireland.

MALCOLM MacLACHLAN lectures in Clinical and Health Psychology at Trinity College Dublin. Dr MacLachlan's major interests concern health promotion, and the role of community and culture in achieving it.

CHAPTER 1

A Healthier Future? An Overview

Eilish Mc Auliffe and Laraine Joyce

Background

Shaping a Healthier Future: a Strategy for Effective Healthcare in the 1990s
(SHF) is one of the most significant policy documents – perhaps *the*
most significant – for the Irish Health Services. It is the culmination
of a series of reports, all suggesting the need for a radical change of
direction in the provision of healthcare in Ireland. The refocusing of
the healthcare system to include health promotion and disease
prevention requires a major shift in our perception of the system's
purpose. The emphasis has broadened from health service planning
to health planning. The focus on outcomes, notably health gain and
social gain for the population, demands that we take stock of what we
are doing and ask the questions that really matter:

- Is the healthcare system having a positive effect on the health of
  the population?
- Are resources being spent to maximum effect?
- How will what we are doing today reflect on the population's
  health in 5–10 years' time?
- Can we plan now to control demand for health services in the future?

This book was born of a curiosity to find out what impact SHF and
the questions it raises are having on managers, clinicians and policy-
makers in our healthcare system. Do they think this change of
direction and refocusing are actually happening in the system, and
what are the critical success factors for healthcare managers in
continuing the change process? Most importantly, we sought opinion
on whether or not the changes in strategy and direction will ultimately
result in a healthier future for the population. Hence, the title of this
book – *A Healthier Future?* – poses the question, 'Are we going in the
right direction?'.

The onus is on healthcare managers and aspiring healthcare managers to take a critical look at the future of healthcare in this country. A considerable number of healthcare management education programmes have been established in the past few years. Students on these programmes will be the policy-makers and managers of the future, and need to learn skills in critical analysis. This book attempts to address the needs of such students. As we near the end of the SHF four-year action plan, it seems important to capture the views and experiences of some of the leading thinkers and key actors in the Irish healthcare system. The book is not meant to be a comprehensive coverage of healthcare management in Ireland, but rather an eclectic mix of views of some key players. To date, there has been a dearth of material that critically analyses the Irish healthcare system. This book aims to address this problem, at least in part.

Content

Part One sets the scene, in terms of setting out what we know about the health status of the Irish population. Health status is defined as a state of complete physical, mental and social well-being. Doorley makes the point that no measures have yet been developed to allow us to measure the health status of a population. Instead we use average lifespan and death rates from particular diseases as indicators of health. SHF has set targets for improvement in health status or health and social gain. Doorley discusses the need for health status indicators in measuring progress on these targets. A public health common data set is being compiled, but the author believes that significant investment is necessary to provide indicators at district level. The indicators that can contribute to some extent in the measurement of health are mentioned. Improvements that have occurred in the health status of the Irish population and progress, in so far as it can be measured, on the targets set out in SHF are discussed. The chapter concludes by highlighting the importance of agreeing baseline health indicators in order to ensure that we can monitor progress on health and social gain targets. In the absence of these baseline indicators, it is difficult to see how we can be assured that a healthier future is in store for the Irish population.

Part Two focuses on the importance of control mechanisms and knowing 'where the buck stops', if we are to ensure that the health services are following the direction set out in SHF. The two chapters in this section argue strongly for greater direction, and the power and authority to move in that direction.

McKevitt argues that in Irish healthcare, the legislative framework is silent on strategy, in contrast to Sweden, Holland and New Zealand, all of which show evidence of measurement and control systems that are tied to specific legislative objectives. In the absence of legislative strategy against which to measure objectives, measurement and accountability become a mechanical and routinised activity: McKevitt argues that this results in the operational driving out the strategic. He further argues that the compliance of managers and professionals in implementing strategy cannot be assumed; it has to be given direction and support through appropriate legislation and the adoption of strategic processes by community-level or street-level public organisations. He concludes that strategy should be seen as consensual and emergent, and less dependent on policy. He also believes that citizen voice needs to be given more attention by what he terms street-level public organisations.

Conroy defines governance as 'authoritative strategic leadership' or 'the exercising of ownership'. He does not believe that Health Boards are currently exercising strategic leadership: 'Boards become over-involved or are passive and claim to be mere volunteers'. He points out that personal and political party goals interfere with the functioning of boards, in the absence of an appropriate job description and model of governance. Conroy perceives the job of a good board as including the following: create ideas; set the mission and values; decide the desired results; look to the future; look to the outside; redefine its mandate; decide the board's floor and the staff's ceiling; separate the wheat from the chaff; set the agenda; and have pride in its work. He argues that policy-making is ends-inspired, and that boards function poorly because they approve means rather than deciding ends.

The accountability legislation, Health (Amendment) (No. 3) Act 1996, addresses to some extent the concerns raised by McKevitt and Conroy, but the focus of this legislation is very much at the top level of the organisation. Where accountability and measurement improve, the healthcare system is dependent on how seriously these concepts are taken on board and cascaded down through the organisation.

Part Three focuses on the funding of healthcare and the fundamental questions that need to be addressed in deciding how to fund, how much to fund, and what to fund. Hederman O'Brien poses the question 'Why spend money on healthcare?'. She suggests that we spend money on healthcare for altruistic reasons and that social solidarity pushes for the strategic organisation of health services.

She goes on to ask 'How should we spend money on healthcare?'. Expert opinion, training of healthcare personnel and research influence this decision. She argues that there is a need for clinicians to become involved in decisions about resource allocation. She suggests a re-examination of training and internship to ensure that the needs of the health system are met. Training in communication skills and management is necessary. She also argues for greater integration of research, development and treatment. Hederman O'Brien gives the example of the Blood Transfusion Service Board and the need to develop transfusion medicine and form links with haematology departments. She highlights the need for an active policy of state-funded research by the Health Research Board in order to ensure that research is integrated in this way, and that it answers the questions 'Why spend money on healthcare?' and 'How should we spend money on healthcare?'.

Lynch examines the trends in healthcare expenditure since the 1960s, and briefly discusses various alternative sources of funding. He points out that the Commission on Health Funding established that there is little to be gained from establishing a separate health fund, i.e. earmarking taxation for health. He argues that to date there is nothing to show how pressure on the public health system could be reduced by an equitable, cost-effective, private-based alternative.

Resource allocation in the Irish healthcare system is moving away from incrementalism to case-mix budgeting which is budget-neutral. He believes that further links between funding and agreed service levels will grow in the future. The chapter concludes by highlighting the challenge of evaluation and its importance in measuring health and social gain and evaluating outcomes of healthcare interventions. The most important question, he says, is not whether enough is being spent on healthcare, but rather what we are achieving with what we are spending.

Brady and West argue that resource management in acute hospitals presents a challenge for all healthcare systems. They draw comparisons between the Irish and UK systems. While acknowledging that the approaches in both systems have met with some success, they believe that the basic problem remains, i.e. that of fixed funds, variable demand, and variations in individual clinicians' practices. They argue that resource management can, however, eliminate some of the inevitable short-term pressures this places on the system, and therefore it needs to be given continued support.

The chapter also highlights the need to specify what treatment should be provided for what patients; otherwise, the authors claim, there will be legitimate scope for variations in clinical practice, and conflicting demands for resources. Brady and West recommend that clear protocols and guidelines be developed and adopted, especially in relation to the quality aspects of care, and argue that clinical leadership is crucial if this process is to succeed. The chapter concludes with a number of issues for decision-makers, on how to ensure that clinical involvement in resource management is effective and how to identify and support clinical leadership.

The contributions of Hederman O'Brien, Lynch, and Brady and West suggest that there is still a long way to go before we can be reassured that we are spending on the most appropriate and cost-effective interventions. The acute hospital services are the primary consumer of resources in our healthcare system. Unless we can manage and control expenditure in secondary and tertiary care, it may be very difficult to achieve the desired balance between treatment and diagnosis on the one hand and health promotion and disease prevention on the other. We cannot continue to throw resources at practices in the absence of information on the effectiveness of those practices.

Part Four addresses the changing nature of the practice of management in the Irish healthcare system. The need to focus on return on investment, or outcomes for inputs; the need to achieve a balance between accountability and risk-taking; the challenge of achieving a higher quality of care at an affordable cost; and the necessity to audit activity and continuously improve quality are highlighted.

Doherty suggests that managers in the public sector must manage for social result, just as managers in the private sector manage for financial result. The public sector must address the bottom-line issue of social return on investment. 'Justification for risk-taking is the social result that will accrue.' He argues that risk management is the entrepreneurial aspect of public management. The Strategic Management Initiative recognises that existing structures and reporting systems promote a risk-averse environment. The transition to a risk-tolerant environment, according to Doherty, requires that civil servants be judged on results and be given discretion in relation to their choice of means.

There is a need to achieve balance between the clinician's accountability to the individual patient and the hospital's account-ability to all taxpayers. Doherty states that three main ideas underpin accountability: advocacy of public values; protection of the public interest; custody of public resources. The Health (Amendment) (No. 3) Act 1996 states that the service plan will form the basis of the accountability relationship between the Chief Executive Officer and the Health Board.

Doherty believes that SHF, new legislation and management development initiatives go a long way towards achieving the balance necessary between encouraging risk-taking and satisfying the accountability expected of the public sector. He concludes by warning that over-emphasis on accountability may create rigidity.

Lynott defines the aim of managed care as being 'to maintain access to high-quality care at an affordable cost'. She suggests that policy-makers and providers need to work together to develop frameworks that will allow the balancing of supply and demand. She feels that the public also have a role in managed care and need to be educated about self-care and prevention, and about the costs of healthcare. Information and clarity of objectives are identified as the foundation of managed care. Lynott argues that the publication of SHF has provided a substantive framework for the planning and delivery of healthcare in Ireland. However, she believes that several issues remain to be addressed before we can hope to achieve managed care, including inter-hospital planning and co-ordination, strengthen-ing management and managing demand and utilisation.

Leahy argues that for any given individual, the only definition of quality that is important is their personal interpretation of the quality of goods and services. However, the professional's view, manager's view, and customer's view must be taken into account. Leahy poses the question 'Why become involved in quality?', and gives several answers to this. In introducing quality initiatives, he points out the need for managers to recognise that resistance to quality is understandable, and says that this resistance may result from difficulty in measuring outcomes, threat to coping mechanisms, i.e. the team approach and camaraderie, or lack of dialogue between disciplines. He suggests two strategies for moving forward:

- development of comparative audit or quality assurance
- initiation of continuous quality improvement, by identifying processes which require multidisciplinary scrutiny. Lessons for managers in conducting audit are that the confidentiality of the doctor–patient relationship must be respected, audit should be adequately resourced and changes implemented, audit is inevitably clinically driven, and managers should cultivate those staff who are committed to audit.

Leahy emphasises the importance of multidisciplinary approaches through the use of quality circles. He also recommends optimising the existing clinical audit programmes and integrating them with other quality assurance systems, establishing quality assurance departments and formalising the involvement of multidisciplinary teams in examining processes.

The contributions of Doherty, Lynott and Leahy highlight the complexity of managing in today's Irish healthcare system. A high calibre of management personnel will be necessary if the balances suggested – between risk-taking and accountability, between cost and quality, and between audit and activity – are to be achieved. These changes are demanding not only on the managers in the system, but also on the very culture of the system. Major culture change is required in order to action the aims of the health strategy. Although this change has begun, it will undoubtedly be a long, slow process, which will be possible only if there is significant focus on the participants in the process. To date, the focus of the strategic change has been on the framework and the services. However, with the establishment of the Office for Health Management and the initiatives it has undertaken to date, the future for the participants (i.e. the managers and potential managers) in our healthcare system looks more hopeful.

Part Five focuses on managing in a multi-agency environment, with particular emphasis on the development of relationships between the statutory and voluntary sectors. In a historical review, Brown argues that the institutionalisation of state hospital policy in the Irish context involved the gradual renegotiation and re-definition of how the public interest and public accountability would best be served. The Hospitals Commission is described as something of a watershed in the evolution of the state's role in, and responsibility for, health services. It confronted directly the role and responsibility of the state for the planning of hospital services for the community. The Commission, although criticised for its bureaucratic approach to the distribution of funds, managed to establish an integrated and publicly accountable system of care for all. This is considered noteworthy, given the institutional diversity, the powerful position and independence of voluntary hospitals and their determination to retain a significant measure of independence. The Commission can also be congratulated for placing greater emphasis on measurement-based accountability, and highlighting the importance of information as a tool in policy-making.

Brown identifies the challenge for hospital managers and planners as the need to achieve a balance between central policy co-ordination (control) and institutional responsiveness and dynamism (autonomy) at the hospital level. She is optimistic that a strong dynamic infrastructure is compatible with an equally strong approach to policy co-ordination. She argues that the development of measurement and information systems can facilitate the co-ordination of policy while allowing greater operating autonomy to hospitals, their managers, professionals and staff.

O'Sullivan states that partnership is important in the health sector, particularly between the statutory and voluntary sectors, since the voluntary sector plays an integral part in the provision of health-care in Ireland. The chapter examines changing relationships between the statutory and voluntary sectors. The author draws our attention to the fact that after a period of neglect, the crisis in the Welfare State has generated an increase in international interest in the voluntary sector. SHF suggested establishing a framework that would recognise the role and responsibilities of both sectors.

A positive justification for the voluntary sector, according to O'Sullivan, is its ability to meet the needs of users in a flexible and effective way. He discusses the concerns each sector may have about the other. The concerns of the statutory sector about the voluntary sector include variations in standards and difficulties of measuring effectiveness, comprehensiveness and co-ordination of services. Voluntary sector concerns include the discretionary nature of funding, the loss of autonomy and lack of influence on planning and policy-making.

O'Sullivan highlights a number of issues that need to be addressed if the voluntary and statutory sectors are to form a partnership. These include putting effective structures in place and drawing up contract/service agreements. He feels strongly that the voluntary sector should be regarded as a very positive reality and resource, and a key strength in our tradition of health service provision in Ireland.

Kenefick raises the concern that the integration of health and social services in Ireland leads to a failure to appreciate the need for somewhat different management approaches and practices in social services. The current 'community care model' necessitates a client-centred approach to service delivery. Some key issues in managing a client-centred community service are discussed, including the need for co-operation between agencies in the multi-agency delivery of a service. The chapter concludes with the essential requirements for managing a decentralised community service.

The voluntary and statutory sectors need to work more closely together, as the Health Boards assume the responsibility for the provision of a comprehensive and integrated service for their catchment populations. Coupled with this is the plan for the Department of Health to transfer the responsibility for funding the voluntary agencies to the Health Boards. With the publication of *Enhancing the Partnership*, an agreement between the Department of Health and the mental handicap agencies, this has become a reality. If this co-ordination and integration is to result in a healthier future for the population, the future relationships between the voluntary and statutory sectors will be crucial.

Part Six argues for the greater involvement of clinicians and professionals in the management of health services, and highlights the support and training needs that should be addressed to encourage this involvement. Joyce stresses the need for clinicians to become involved in the management of health services. She discusses the reasons for the reluctance of some clinicians to become involved. This arises partly from the clash that can occur between the managerial and the medical culture. The results of a recent survey of consultants and senior registrars on their perceived management training needs are presented. The data are comparable to those of a similar survey in the UK. A surprisingly high proportion of Irish consultants stated that they already had significant management responsibilities. Senior registrars appeared to be more interested in assuming a managerial role, and more of them had received some form of management training, which may augur well for the future involvement of doctors in management.

Joyce argues for a unidisciplinary approach to training for doctors initially, and points out the importance of flexibility in scheduling training events. She also suggests the use initially of training styles with which the doctors are familiar and comfortable, i.e. the more didactic styles, and that they should build on the existing concerns and interests. For doctors who are to assume a more active managerial and clinical leadership role she advocates multidisciplinary approaches to training and team-building, particularly where new management structures are being developed and trust needs to be engendered.

McCarthy suggests that leadership in Irish nursing needs to be strengthened and points out that transformational leaders are required to achieve this aim. Transformational leaders are innovative and evolutionary and develop trust through decentralisation and participation. Transactional leaders, by contrast, are concerned with completing the task at hand and maintaining the *status quo*. McCarthy argues that Irish nurse leaders have in the main been the products of autocratic systems, and mentored into using transactional styles. Leaders of the past have shaped a culture which socialised nurses into deferential roles.

She argues that it is important to match the nurse to the job, and not push nurses into leadership roles in cases where they are obtaining job satisfaction at front-line level. A three-tiered structure of nursing is proposed, with the work at director level being strategic and the work at divisional and first line operational. As the roles of nurse managers evolve, education and training in leadership need to be provided. The implementation of SHF requires devolving accountability and the involvement of nurses in management at all levels.

Since the completion of McCarthy's chapter, the interim report of the Commission on Nursing has been published, and also highlights issues of leadership and management in nursing and notes initiatives being taken by the Office for Health Management to address some of these issues.

Part Seven focuses on the recipients of healthcare and those whose needs the healthcare system is charged with serving. The argument is for greater involvement of citizens in the healthcare of their communities, and a greater involvement of patients/consumers of healthcare in the design and planning of services.

Kevany makes the point that the democratisation of public-sector planning, progressive decentralisation of administrative and budgetary functions, greater public interest in health issues, and the rise in costs of care systems all demand a new approach to the way that primary care systems are designed and operated. It is argued that to ensure both effectiveness and efficiency, services should respond as closely as possible to communities' perceptions of need and expectations of response. The chapter argues strongly for community participation, defined as 'substantive and continuous involvement of the community in the design, management and resourcing of its primary care system'. Kevany discusses the benefits of community participation and high-lights the main steps or components in the process. Reference is made to some community participation projects that have met with success in Ireland.

The Government document *A Health Promotion Strategy* is subtitled *Making the Healthier Choice the Easier Choice*. MacLachlan argues that in many Irish contexts the healthier choice is far from the easier choice. He draws attention, in particular, to travellers, and states that attempts to assimilate travellers into the existing health services have sometimes been culturally insensitive. The Primary Health Care for Travellers Project has attempted to overcome this insensitivity by developing a distinctive profile of travellers' health and involving travellers in the promotion of health. MacLachlan also discusses the community reactions in inner city Dublin to its drug problems, and suggests that these reactions should not be viewed simply as preventive or curative, but should be recognised as a response that has the potential to be actively health-promoting. He refers to the Kilkenny Health project and the need for community involvement and a bottom-up approach to health promotion.

The components of the different contexts in which health pro-motion must be effective are also considered, e.g. the influence of poverty, urban–rural differences and the Irish culture. MacLachlan urges healthcare managers to pay greater attention to the social contexts of health problems and to recognise that target groups may have the potential to develop their own solutions. In conclusion, he states that in order to make the healthier choice the easier choice,

11

'health promotion efforts must incorporate cultural, community and contextual resources that are available to us'.

Mc Auliffe briefly examines the concept of patient-centred care, as well as the developments in acknowledging the rights of the consumer. It is argued that restructuring services to achieve patient-centred care is not sufficient in itself. The voice of the consumer must be heard if we are truly to achieve patient-centred care. The concept of the 'consumer' is explored – who are they, why should we involve them, and (on the continuum between consultation and active partici-pation) how involved do we want them to become? Techniques for involving consumers are discussed and examples provided. The chapter concludes with a framework for planning consumer involvement, and strongly recommends that managers adopt this in order to avoid the frequent pitfalls in this field. She calls for a national effort to encourage the involvement of citizens in healthcare planning and decision-making, and points out that this is the one dimension of the health strategy that has not been addressed to date by the Department of Health.

The contributions of Kevany, MacLachlan, and Mc Auliffe all provide examples of community involvement in healthcare. However, much remains to be done in gaining widespread involvement of communities in identifying their health needs and in designing and planning services that respond to these needs. Mc Auliffe points out that this is the one dimension of SHF that has not been directly addressed by the Department of Health to date. We cannot ignore the escalating litigation cases in healthcare. If the aim is to get citizens to take responsibility for their own healthcare, there is a need to encourage and support their education on, and involvement in, healthcare.

The way forward

A question was posed at the outset – 'Are we going in the right direction?'. What conclusions can be drawn from the above com-pilation of views?

The consensus emerging from the authors' contributions is that yes, we are going in the right direction. All the chapters support the ideas and principles contained in SHF. It is useful to recall that the Irish health service is not being reformed – it is being 'reshaped'. Healthcare reform in Ireland is thus a rather stealthy and incremental process. Progress has therefore been slow. It has the significant advantage, however, that the national health strategy has been endorsed by successive governments, and supported by all major political parties.

SHF is not imbued with any strong pro-market philosophy. Rather, the intent is to maintain the strong caring ethos in the Irish health system and try to marry that with the best in the new public management.

In essence, the Irish approach to reform has been to streamline existing structures, devolve more decision-making to a regional level and tighten up on managerial accountability and performance. But whether or not there are sufficient incentives and sanctions in the current system to encourage real and lasting change remains to be seen.

Managers, for instance, are mostly appointed on a permanent basis, although this is changing for some new appointments. There are no systems of performance appraisal or performance management in operation as yet. If there were, they would be hampered by a lack of management information. At present, there are limited links between activity and funding for hospitals, although this is changing with the increasing use of case-mix data.

Hospital consultants, who have significant influence, have currently little incentive to become involved in the hospital management process. Nevertheless, the number of doctors expressing an interest in management is likely to grow in the future.

Another potential block to change is the level of investment in managers themselves. Traditionally, there has been no major investment in management development, and managerial salary levels are low in comparison with northern Europe. General management is not well developed.

The constraints on public expenditure, and on health spending in particular, are not likely to diminish. It is difficult to see how spending in the acute sector is to be contained in the future. We may yet have to adopt a more radical strategy in order to manage care more effectively. This will require the establishment of a strong general management function, personnel packages that give managers the incentive to manage through fixed-term contracts and performance management systems, and a much increased investment in management training and development.

The demand from the centre is for greater accountability and a more outcome-focused, performance-based service. Service planning is to be the cornerstone of that change, yet it remains unproven.

Key to the new accountability will be the implementation of the new legislation, the Health (Amendment) (No. 3) Act 1996. Underlying this is the need to control costs in the acute sector. That will require the real involvement of doctors in the management process, the introduction of new hospital management structures to accommodate that involvement, and the more skilled use of existing information at hospital level.

The ingredients for a reshaped and revitalised health service are on the table. Progress has been slow, but it has been in the right direction. What is needed now is for managers and policy-makers to lead, and not just manage, the process of shaping a health service for the twenty-first century. The vision of the authors is that this must be a health service that focuses on outcomes and results, is consumer-oriented and outward looking, facilitates team working, values diversity and encourages local innovation and risk-taking within a framework of accountability.

PART ONE

The Health Status of the Irish Population

CHAPTER 2

Health Status

Patrick Doorley

What is health status?

Good health is defined as a 'state of complete physical, mental, and social well-being'. Health status refers to the present state of illness or 'wellness' in a community, and can be described in terms of rates of death and illness in a community, the prevalence of good and poor health practices, rates of death and disease (chronic and infectious) and the prevalence of symptoms/conditions of well-being.

Determinants of health

Many factors influence individual and population health, most of which are outside the control of the health services. The main influences are:

- genetic factors which determine an individual's predisposition to disease
- environmental factors such as air and water pollution and housing
- lifestyle factors such as smoking, alcohol use, exercise and diet
- socio-economic factors.

Measurement of health status

There is no single 'standard' measurement of health status for individuals or population groups. Individual health status may be measured by an observer (e.g. a physician), who performs an examination and rates the individual along any of several dimensions, including the presence or absence of life-threatening illness, risk factors for premature death, severity of disease, and overall health. Individual health status may also be assessed by asking the person to report his/her health perceptions in certain areas, such as physical functioning, emotional well-being, pain or discomfort, and overall perception of health. Although it is theoretically attractive to argue that the measurement of health should consist of the combination of an objective component and the individual's subjective impressions, no such measure has been developed.

The health of an entire population is determined by aggregating data collected on individuals. The health of an individual is easier to define than the health of a population. Once the definition of optimum health for the individual is agreed upon, health status can be placed along a continuum from perfect health to death. No comparable scale exists for whole populations.

In the absence of comprehensive or absolute measures of the health of a population, the average lifespan, the death rates from specific diseases, the prevalence of specific diseases, and availability of health services serve as indicators of health status. Judgements regarding the level of health of a particular population are usually made by comparing one population with another, or by studying the trends in a health indicator within a population over time.

The Health Strategy document, *Shaping a Healthier Future*, brought the concepts of health gain and social gain to the fore in the Irish health services for the first time. The Health Strategy discusses progress which has been made on some of the more important health indicators in Ireland over the past few decades, and sets targets for improvement in the health status of the Irish population over the next decade or so. The remainder of this chapter discusses the need for health status indicators, the different indicators that can contribute to the measurement of health status, improvements that have occurred in the health status of the Irish population, and the prospects for further improvements.

Why do we need health status indicators?

- Health status indicators can be used to compare the health status of different populations between and within countries.
- They can help the process of setting goals and priorities.
- They can indicate what progress we are making in improving the health of the population.
- They give an indication of the health needs of the population and, to a lesser extent, health service needs.

Public health common data set

Many countries have drawn up what is termed a 'public health common data set'. This attempts to depict the health status of the population using different dimensions. The data sets used are usually detailed, but the main categories of information include:

- life expectancy
- death rates – overall death rates, and death rates for specific diseases, e.g. cancers and heart disease, with rates standardised for age and sex to allow comparison between demographically different populations
- morbidity data – the incidence and prevalence of specific diseases, e.g. coronary heart disease, arthritis and AIDS
- patterns of lifestyle, e.g. information on smoking habits, diet, exercise, alcohol abuse and drug abuse
- self-perceived health from validated questionnaires such as the SF36 questionnaire.

While improvements in health cannot be entirely or largely attributable to healthcare interventions, we must monitor trends in health and in the factors which influence health if we are to know what progress we are making. At the time of writing, some of the more important elements of the Irish public health common data set are just becoming available for the first time, e.g. standardised mortality rates for many causes of death, by Health Board and by county. However, a significant investment in health information will be required in order to provide data at district electoral division (DED) level.

Geographical variations in health status

The health indicators mentioned above, if available on a small-area basis (i.e. at ward or DED level), can be used to highlight differences in the health experience of people living in different geographical areas. So far in Ireland, the availability of such data is limited almost entirely to the Eastern Health Board area. Small-area health information can be useful for the following reasons.

- It may help in identifying areas where health indicators are poor, so that special interventions can be targeted at the populations concerned.

- It may help to answer questions about alleged high incidence or prevalence of diseases such as cancer, and in some cases may help to identify possible causes of disease and death.
- It may help to evaluate the impact of special health interventions targeted at specific areas. Bear in mind the caveat entered above in relation to attribution of health status improvement to specific interventions. A control area of roughly similar health, socio-economic and demographic status may help to overcome this difficulty.

Life expectancy

Life expectancy at birth is one of the most important health status indicators for population groups. Life expectancy at birth is not simply the average age at which people die – it is a more complex and hypothetical statistic. It is calculated by applying the death rates within each five-year or one-year age group, and within each sex from the population under study, to a hypothetical birth cohort of 100,000 individuals. Lower life expectancy in developing countries is usually a result of high infant mortality. Life expectancy in Ireland, at 72.8 years for men and 78 years for women, is a little below the average for the European Union. If we use life expectancy at the age of 40, the comparison is more unfavourable, with Irish women doing worst and Irish men second-worst of all countries in the European Union.

In most countries, improvement in average life expectancy at birth comes initially from improvements in infant mortality. There is some correlation of average life expectancy at birth with average expenditure per capita on health, but there is probably a stronger correlation with GDP per capita. Since many factors influence average life expectancy in a population, differences between different countries cannot neatly be attributed to one or two factors. However, the Health Strategy does acknowledge that Ireland's high rates of deaths from cardiovascular diseases and certain cancers are important contributory factors. Life expectancy at birth continues to improve in most EU countries, and the overall objective set in the Health Strategy is to improve Irish life expectancy so as to move over time to the higher levels prevailing in other EU countries.

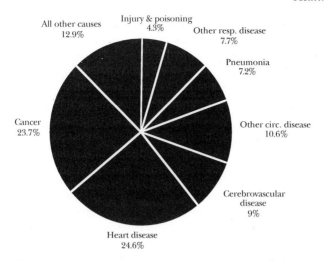

Fig. 2.1. Principal causes of death (percentage distribution), 1995

Causes of death

Principal causes of death

Figure 2.1 shows deaths in Ireland by principal causes for the year 1995. Cardiovascular diseases, which include the categories of heart disease and diseases of the blood vessels (mostly strokes) and other circulatory diseases, account for approximately 44% of deaths. Cancer accounts for approximately 24%. However, because older people feature disproportionately among the deaths from cardiovascular diseases, when we come to look at causes of premature deaths (deaths under the age of 65), cancer becomes the most important cause, accounting for 33%, followed by cardiovascular disease at 29%, with accidents being the third most common specific cause of premature death. The importance of accidental death would therefore be greatly reduced if we simply looked at deaths among all age groups.

Mortality rates

Death rates (mortality data) form the basis for assessing the health status of the population. Mortality rates can be calculated for deaths by all causes combined, by specific causes, and by particular age–sex groups. In order to compare mortality rates across different populations, groups or time periods, the rates must be 'standardised' to a population with the same age structure. The UK population, for example, has an older age structure then the Irish population. We would expect therefore that crude (non-standardised) death rates might be higher in the UK. In order to make a valid comparison, the death rates for each country must be adjusted to a common population with a known age structure. When reviewing mortality statistics, therefore, always check whether you are looking at standardised or crude mortality rates. Even these adjustments, however, do not take full account of important causes of mortality which have a greater that average impact on middle-aged and younger people, e.g. deaths from accidents. Thus one finds that the measure known as years of potential life lost (YPLL) is becoming increasingly popular (Centers for Disease Control, 1997). YPLL is considered in some quarters to be a policy-relevant indicator by comparison with crude or age-standardised death rates, because it can produce a different ranking of the major causes of death. For example, accidents may be ranked low as a cause of death in a country in terms of standardised mortality rates (SMRs); on the basis of YPLL accidents may become much more significant.

'Avoidable deaths' can be a performance indicator as well as a health status indicator. An avoidable death can be defined as a death from a condition amenable to medical intervention. The European Community atlas of 'avoidable death' (Holland, 1991, 1993) has recently received prominence, given international recognition of the need to develop measures of the outcome of healthcare services, as well as indices of need for health services. If an avoidable death is not avoided, there are a number of potential causes: for instance, resources may not be available, the organisation of health services may be inefficient or inappropriate, or professional practice may be sub-optimal.

As indicators of health in developed countries, mortality data have the advantage of universality and long historical continuity. Despite the problem of changes in diagnostic and classification practices, they are the most reliable of the health status indicators. However, in a country like Ireland, where overall health status is high by international standards, death rates alone are no longer an adequate measure of population health. Increasing numbers of health problems are emerging which do not threaten life but are responsible for substantial amounts of continuing ill-health and disability. Health expectancy – a composite health indicator which takes life expectancy and breaks it down into years of disability-free and disabled life – is being used increasingly in other countries to take account of the rising prevalence of chronic illness in the face of increased longevity. This indicator is not yet available in Ireland, but is one which should form part of the public health common data set.

Morbidity data

Information about non-fatal but chronic disabling illnesses can be gained from hospital admission statistics, from disease notifications, from special registers of illness and disability and from the results of health surveys and special epidemiological studies. These sources, some of which are discussed below, can provide more sensitive and timely indicators of public health than can mortality data, but each has its limitations when used in this way.

Reported morbidity (illness) rates are much less reliable than mortality data, as their collection and collation depend on people making contact with the health services. They are therefore more properly indicators of health services utilisation. It is well known, for example, that elderly people who need treatment often do not seek it as they presume that the conditions that affect them are simply part of growing old. However, robust data collected by general practitioners on the reasons for consultation can be useful, especially if they are collected as part of a sentinel practice survey system, where there is good quality control.

The Hospital In-Patient Enquiry System (HIPE) gives information on all discharges from acute hospitals, but these data are more a reflection of utilisation of that hospital's service than an indicator of morbidity in the community.

Infectious diseases are notifiable, but it is generally accepted that notification is very incomplete. These data are therefore used as an indication more of trends than of the actual incidence or prevalence of disease in the community.

Registers of disability can be very useful in the assessment of needs for services. In the past few years in Ireland a National Register of Intellectual Disability has been established in each Health Board area, and a register of physical disability is to be piloted. Special registers of certain conditions can give a good idea of the incidence and prevalence of these conditions, e.g. coronary heart disease, stroke and diabetes. Such registers require ongoing maintenance and are costly. Registers for these important conditions do not exist in Ireland. We do, however, have a National Cancer Registry. The National Cancer Registry is a very useful source of data on cancer incidence. Looking at cancer deaths from the Central Statistics Office (CSO) data and comparing them with cancer incidence from the National Cancer Registry, one can see that in the case of those cancers which are almost invariably fatal within a short period, e.g. lung cancer, cancer deaths almost equal cancer incidence. With cancers where survival is better, e.g. breast cancer, the number of deaths might be equal to about half the number of cases per year. In the long term, therefore, cancer registries can help to give an indication of survival and therefore of the effectiveness of medical treatment. At some time in the future, it will be possible to get data on cancer incidence on a small-area basis, e.g. the incidence in each ward or DED. When a number of years of such data have been accumulated, they may help answer questions about possible associations between environmental hazards and alleged increased rates of cancer in localised areas.

Health-related quality of life

A number of questionnaires have been designed in order to measure health-related quality of life (HRQL) in individuals and populations. Some of these are disease-specific, while others are more general quality-of-life instruments. The latter include the Nottingham Health Profile, Euroquol and SF36. SF36 has been most widely used and validated among populations. SF36 is in fact a short form of a much more detailed medical outcomes study (MOS) questionnaire. It measures the eight most important of the 40 concepts measured in the MOS. SF36 is a practical and valid instrument for measuring health status and outcomes from the patient's point of view. Designed for use in surveys of general and specific populations, health policy evaluations and clinical practice and research, the survey can be self-administered by people 14 years of age and older, or administered by trained interviewers either in person or by telephone. SF36 measures the following eight health concepts, which are relevant across age, disease and treatment groups:

- limitations in physical activities because of health problems
- limitations in usual role activities because of physical health

- bodily pain
- general health perceptions
- vitality (energy and fatigue)
- limitations in social activities because of physical or emotional problems
- limitations in usual role activities because of emotional problems
- mental health (psychological distress and well-being).

The survey's standardised scoring system yields a profile of eight health scores, a self-evaluated change in health status, and physical and mental health summary measures.

SF36 has been normed in the general US population and for representative samples in Denmark, Germany, Sweden and the UK. It has been used on a very limited basis in Ireland, mainly in studies assessing the improvement in the quality of life for patients who have had particular interventions.

Euroquol, another general health status instrument, based on six different dimensions of general health, was developed by the International Euroquol Group. In developing this instrument, the group found striking similarities in relative valuations attached to different health status of people in England, the Netherlands and Sweden. Other instruments used internationally include the Nottingham Health Profile and the Rand General Health Perception Questionnaire. Despite increasing use, particularly in economic studies, no 'gold standard' exists.

No 'gold standard' exists for the measurement of HRQL in populations. A lot more work needs to be done in order to ensure that HRQL instruments will be used with the same confidence that other health indicators command at present.

National Health Strategy targets related to the main causes of death

Cardiovascular diseases

Although heart disease death rates for both men and women have been falling in Ireland over the past two decades, the standardised death rates for both men and women are more than twice as high as the EU average. Some authors have linked the decline in mortality from ischaemic heart disease in different countries to better treatment of high blood pressure. Others have attributed at least part of the decline to direct treatment of ischaemic heart disease. The consensus is that 60% of the decline was due to changes in lifestyle and the remainder to medical care. The standardised death rate from strokes has decreased dramatically over the past few decades, and is now around the EU average.

The important risk factors relating to death rates from cardio-vascular disease include smoking (which accounts for approximately 25% of ischaemic heart disease), high blood cholesterol (which is to some extent linked to the fat content of the diet), lack of physical exercise, and untreated high blood pressure.

Prospects for achieving strategy target: The medium-term target is to reduce the death rate from cardiovascular disease in the under 65 age group by 30% over ten years. In order to achieve this, there will have to be further reductions in smoking prevalence and the prevalence of high cholesterol, and improvements in the treatment of high blood pressure and in the level of physical activity of the population. The treatment of established heart disease, including acute events, will also have an important contribution to make. In this respect, it has been shown that more widespread use of potentially life-saving anti-clotting agents within hours of a heart attack has the potential to reduce early deaths from heart attacks. The contribution to health gain from coronary artery bypass surgery (CABG) consists mainly of improvements in the quality of life. Although there is an increased life expectancy among certain subgroups, the contribution which other procedures such as angioplasty can make has yet to be fully evaluated. It should be possible to achieve the Health Strategy target on cardiovascular diseases, but much will depend on the progress we make in tackling the major risk factors.

Cancer

From present trends, it is anticipated that overall mortality in the European Union will increase over the next 15 years in the absence of more effective strategies for prevention and treatment. While Ireland's death rate from cancer has declined by almost 10% in the under 65 age group since 1970, it is still above the EU average and our mortality rate for the overall population (i.e. including those over 65) has been rising slightly since the late 1970s.

The main sources of our above-average mortality compared with the EU are cancers of the lung, breast, and colon and rectum. Male deaths in Ireland from lung cancer have been falling, but mortality from this cause is increasing among women. As it takes about 15 to 20 years for tobacco to induce lung cancer, these mortality rates reflect smoking patterns among men and women 15 to 20 years ago. Deaths from both colorectal cancer and breast cancer have risen slightly in recent years.

In 1996, the Department of Health produced a cancer strategy which included the following commitments.

- Research will be undertaken into the causes of the apparent variations in cancer incidents and mortality between different parts of the country.
- Health promotion will form a key element of an integrated approach to the strategy.
- Screening and early detection programmes will form a critical part of the drive to combat cancer mortality and morbidity.
- Cancer treatment services will be reorganised using an integrated model of primary and hospital care.
- Regional directors of cancer services will be appointed and will prepare a plan for the development of cancer services in their region (Department of Health, 1996a).

Prospects for achieving Health Strategy targets: Research suggests that the management of cancer and its outcomes can be improved if care is provided by specialists working in multidisciplinary teams with a sufficient throughput of new cases per year. The full implementation of the National Cancer Strategy should therefore help to improve the outcomes for treatment of cancer in Ireland. However, it must be borne in mind that even with well-organised services giving treatment according to the best protocols, survival rates for many of the common cancers are still quite low, e.g. the five-year survival rate for cancer of the lung is less than 10%, that for cancer of the stomach less than 20%, that for cancer of the colon less than 50%. The greatest improvements in survival have been achieved in the treatment of leukaemias among children. By tackling problems like smoking, alcohol abuse and poor diet, we could prevent a very significant number of cancers. However, the benefits of some of these interventions will not be seen within ten years. For these reasons, the targets relating to prevention of cancer deaths will be more difficult to achieve.

Accidents

Accidental injury is identified in the Health Strategy as one of the three major causes of premature death in Ireland. Because so many deaths from accidental injury occur in young or middle-aged people, it is the single greatest cause of years of potential life lost before the age of 65 and is a major reason for disability in all age groups. The Health Strategy acknowledges that there has been a reduction in accidental deaths of 37% over the past 20 years. The death rate in Ireland for injury is significantly lower than the EU average. Because it is necessary to work with many other agencies in order to make significant progress, no target has been set in the Strategy for reduction in deaths from accidental injury pending consultation with the relevant agencies.

In 1996 the Office for Health Gain published a report, *Accidental Injury in Ireland – Priorities for Prevention*, which highlighted the following facts.

- Over 500,000 Irish people each year require treatment as a result of accidents.
- 55,000 of these need to be admitted to hospital.
- Accidents account for over 40% of all deaths in children and over one-third of deaths up to the age of 45 years.
- Accidents are a cause of much illness and disability.
- Most accidents can be prevented.

There is much evidence to suggest that the health services could achieve better outcomes by improving pre-hospital treatment (e.g. by having well-trained paramedics who can perform advanced resuscitation), by improved treatment of certain conditions such as multiple serious injuries and by putting more emphasis on rehabilitation. However, there is probably even more potential health gain to be achieved through prevention. This requires co-operation with other agencies.

The Office for Health Gain has taken a lead in establishing a National Accident Forum whose aim is to facilitate a co-ordinated approach to accident prevention at national and regional level. The Forum set priorities for 1997 as follows:

- reducing accidents among small children in the home
- reducing falls in the elderly
- developing better information systems.

Information systems: High-quality and timely information is essential in order to plan for better accident prevention. At present the main data sources are the Central Statistics Office, Hospital In-patient Enquiry System and National Roads Authority. These tend to capture serious injuries. At present most Accident and Emergency Departments cannot turn their large quantities of data on injuries into useful information. Thus, information on approximately 90% of all injuries is not available. The Forum aims to work with the relevant disciplines towards developing an injury information system.

Although accidents are identified as one of the three main causes of premature death in Ireland, there is no Health Strategy target as yet. Progress will depend on the performance of many different agencies, and is therefore difficult to predict.

Risk factors for disease

Most countries include population data or risk factors for major diseases as part of their public health common data set. The Health Strategy lists six areas in which risk reduction targets and action programmes are to be focused. These are discussed below in terms of the *status quo* as we know it, the progress that has been made and opportunities for further improvement.

Smoking

Smoking is by far the single greatest cause of preventable death in Ireland today. It causes 6,000 deaths each year, which is more than the combined total for alcohol, drugs, AIDS, accidents and suicide. Smoking causes 90% of cases of lung cancer, about 25% of cases of coronary heart disease, and contributes significantly to other fatal illnesses such as chronic bronchitis and a number of other cancers. The Health Strategy target is to reduce the prevalence of smoking among adults to 20% by the year 2000. The prevalence of smoking among adults has fallen from the mid-1970s level of around 45% to the current level of 28%. However, the decline has slowed up in recent years, and in fact there has been no change since the Health Strategy target was set three years ago. Furthermore, there is concern about high levels of smoking among young people. The Health Strategy target was an ambitious one, and it appears now that it is unlikely to be achieved. When smoking prevalence drops below 30%, it becomes more difficult to make further progress. However, even a modest decline in smoking prevalence would produce a level of health gain in future years which would not be achieved even from large investments in other areas of the health service. The international evidence suggests that a combination of very strong policy measures is needed in order to achieve further progress. The most important of these would be the following.

- Fiscal measures, e.g. continued increases in taxation well above the level of inflation with a provision for some of this taxation to be earmarked for purposes of health promotion. Fiscal measures are the most important in terms of achieving progress in the short term. They also have a greater impact on young people.
- A total ban on tobacco advertising and sponsorship. This is particularly important in relation to children's smoking, as it has been shown that children are aware of, remember and are influenced by tobacco advertising.

Progress: Ireland has in the past given a lead in the area of health policy by introducing certain measures which were later adopted as standard EU practice, e.g. health warnings on cigarette packages. Since the publication of the Health Strategy the legislation on smoking in public places has been strengthened. There have been increases in taxation on cigarettes which have been around or slightly above the level of inflation. In line with Department of Health policy, the allowable budgets for advertising and sponsorship have been reduced by 5% per annum. The Office for Health Gain has initiated a number of campaigns: for example, one campaign aimed at discouraging the illegal sale of cigarettes to children, and other campaigns have highlighted the dangers of passive smoking and encouraged the provision of smoke-free public places. However, it is disappointing that the three years after the publication of the Health Strategy document represents a period in which no progress has been made on one of the most important targets of the Health Strategy. There now needs to be an urgent review with a view to strengthening policy, particularly in the areas mentioned above.

Alcohol

The average consumption of alcohol per head of population has more than doubled since 1960. In any country there is a clear and direct relationship between the extent of alcohol consumption and alcohol-related problems. Although many European countries have a higher per capita consumption of alcohol, alcohol-related problems are a major public health problem in Ireland.

The number of deaths from alcohol is more difficult to quantify than that from smoking. However, alcohol plays an important role in many deaths in Ireland each year. Alcohol is causally related to cancers of the digestive tract and the liver, and contributes to high blood pressure, cirrhosis of the liver, and deaths from road traffic accidents and suicide. The level of spouse abuse, child abuse and other violence related to alcohol is difficult to quantify but is undoubtedly highly significant. The number of deaths from cirrhosis of the liver has shown a slight upward trend in the past ten years. However, this, like the other diseases associated with alcohol, is not a highly specific indicator. Admissions to psychiatric hospitals for alcohol disorders have decreased in recent years, but there has undoubtedly been a major increase in the number of people being treated in alternative centres, for which we do not have figures.

Health Strategy: The Health Strategy identified alcohol consumption as a key risk factor which contributes to the three main causes of premature death in Ireland (heart disease, cancer and accidents). The Health Strategy objective is to promote moderation in the consumption of alcohol and to reduce the risks to physical, mental and family health that can arise from alcohol abuse. The target is to ensure that within four years, 75% of the adult population should know and understand the recommended sensible limits for alcohol consumption. The recommended limits are 14 units of alcohol per week for a woman and 21 units a week for a man.

National Alcohol Policy: In 1996, the Department of Health produced a National Alcohol Policy (Department of Health, 1996b). Among the areas identified for action were the following:

- promoting awareness of sensible drinking guidelines
- professional training
- education on alcohol in schools
- voluntary identity card schemes
- workplace alcohol policies
- access to alcohol
- alcohol pricing
- treatment services.

The National Alcohol Policy recognises that alcohol consumption is set to increase in the Irish population in the coming years, for a number of reasons:

- the current and projected economic growth
- an anticipated increase in the number of people drinking more beer which is less sensitive to price increases
- possible greater access to alcohol through longer opening hours
- a greater number of young people starting to drink at a younger age
- strong alcohol advertising campaigns and sponsorship campaigns.

Progress: In 1995, Ireland, along with 48 other states, adopted the European Charter on Alcohol, which advocates strong multisectoral policies on alcohol. It is extremely important, just as in the case of smoking, that we should have a comprehensive package of strong policy measures which would include severe restrictions, if not a total ban, on alcohol advertising, and regular increases in taxation of alcohol above the level of inflation. In the absence of such policies, alcohol consumption and alcohol-related problems are likely to rise in Ireland in the years ahead. In this respect, it is disappointing that for the third time in a row, the 1997 budget failed to produce any increase in taxation on alcohol. This may well reflect a certain ambivalence among policy-makers as well as among the general public on the question of alcohol in Ireland. It is unlikely, therefore, that progress in this area will be made until the policy measures outlined in the National Alcohol Strategy are implemented.

Nutrition and diet

Nutrition is an important influence on two of the three causes of premature death in Ireland, namely cardiovascular disease and cancer. In addition, nutrition has a very significant bearing on the development of osteoporosis, diabetes mellitus and obesity. These are conditions which are relatively common and of great significance to the health services. The specific targets are:

- to reduce the average fat intake to no more than 35% of energy by the year 2005, and to achieve an appropriate balance of fats in the diet
- to achieve a reduction of 10 percentage points in the percentage

of the population who are overweight by the year 2005

- to achieve a reduction of 10 percentage points in the percentage of people who are obese by the year 2005.

The data currently available on Irish dietary habits are not adequate. A National Study conducted by the Irish National Dietetics Institute (INDI) in 1990 showed that in certain age groups the fat content of the diet was too high. 53% of adult men and 33% of adult women were found to be overweight, with an additional 10% of males and 15% of females classified as obese. The high fat content of the Irish diet is particularly important in view of our high rates of coronary heart disease (CHD) and bowel cancer. Obesity is a recognised risk factor for CHD, and overall mortality is higher in those who are overweight.

Other information on Irish dietary patterns comes from the Kilkenny Health Project surveys of 1985 and 1990, The Happy Heart survey 1992 and the Health Works Project 1993. The information from these surveys suggests that compared to our European neighbours, we are relatively low consumers of fruit and vegetables and fish. It appears that people are tending to decrease their fat consumption, but further improvement in this area is desirable. The 1990 INDI survey was the most comprehensive survey of dietary patterns in Ireland for many years, but the information it yielded was not complete. It is important that we now have a comprehensive dietary survey which will give us all the information we need about dietary patterns in Ireland today.

The Department of Health developed a Framework for Action on Nutrition in 1991. This includes a series of healthy eating guidelines which have been very visibly and successfully promoted each year for the past few years in conjunction with the food industries in Healthy Eating Week. A National Nutrition Surveillance Centre has been established in the Health Promotion Department of UCG. A successful peer-led intervention programme has been conducted by the Eastern Health Board in conjunction with the Department of Health in one of the more deprived areas of Dublin. This might serve as a model for other parts of the country. However, the Health Boards have only a small fraction of the complement of community nutritionists which would allow them to conduct programmes promoting healthy eating in the community. There is therefore a serious resource constraint on the implementation of the Framework for Action on Nutrition.

Progress: Although it appears that the Irish diet is becoming healthier, we currently do not have sufficient information. The INDI study mentioned above unfortunately did not yield sufficient information to give a comprehensive baseline. There is good reason to believe that the Irish dietary pattern will continue to improve, but we urgently need a comprehensive study which will give a good baseline against which we can measure future progress.

Cholesterol

The blood level of cholesterol is generally accepted as a very important risk factor for coronary heart disease. The baseline survey of the Kilkenny Health Project, which is often taken as a proxy for the rest of the country, indicated that a majority of middle-aged adults had a level of cholesterol which was too high. The target for cholesterol set out in the Health Promotion Strategy document (Department of Health, 1995b) is that mean cholesterol among Irish adults will be lowered from its current level of 5.6 to 5.2 (the evidence suggests that the benefit of lowering cholesterol much below 5.2 is not great). This implies that the majority of adults in Ireland could lower their risk of coronary heart disease by lowering their cholesterol levels. However, population screening for cholesterol levels is not generally recommended. As the blood cholesterol level is to some extent related to diet, a more pragmatic approach is:

- to encourage general practitioners to screen those whom they consider to be at high risk, e.g. close relatives of patients who have developed coronary heart disease at an early age
- to promote the Department of Health's Healthy Eating Guidelines among the general population.

A very aggressive approach towards the detection and management of high cholesterol has been taken in the United States, and this may be one of the reasons why deaths rates from coronary heart disease in the United States are lower than those in Ireland. The prospects for medical treatment of those with very high cholesterol levels appear to have improved in recent years. The increasing number of practice nurses attached to general practices in Ireland should facilitate general practitioners in conducting work of this kind. However, many will point to the fact that health promotion by general practitioners in the United Kingdom has not been an unqualified success. The likelihood is that, with improving dietary patterns and better detection and treatment for high cholesterol, the average cholesterol levels will decrease over the next decade or so.

Physical exercise

The most recent and wide-ranging study on involvement in physical activity in Ireland was conducted in 1991 by the Health Promotion Unit in partnership with the Department of Education. The key finding in this study was that only 53% of 16–75-year-olds participate once a week or more often in some physical activity. Physical activity levels decline with age in both sexes, with men generally more active than women. Walking is the most popular activity, followed by swimming and cycling. Reasons for participating were mainly related to health, enjoyment and socialisation. Not enough time, lack of facilities, and expense were the three top reasons why people did not become involved in sport and physical activities.

The Kilkenny Health Project found that only one quarter of adults participated in 'heart healthy activity', i.e. physical exercise of sufficient intensity and frequency to give a protective effect against coronary heart disease. The Happy Heart survey found that 22% of respondents were sedentary, 54% undertook light activities, while only 25% were involved in vigorous activities. A study in the Eastern Health Board area in 1990 showed that overall, only 22% of the young middle-aged adult population participated in 'heart healthy' activities.

The level of physical activity among the Irish population is low, although it is not markedly different to the situation in the UK and the United States.

Benefits of exercise: Moderate and regular exercise leads to improved heart function and increased strength of muscles and ligaments, while vigorous regular exercise substantially reduces the risk of coronary heart disease. Weight-bearing exercise (not swimming or cycling) helps to prevent osteoporosis. Exercise also helps to reduce anxiety/depression and may improve self-confidence and self-esteem.

Provisional targets in relation to exercise were set out in the Health Strategy as follows:

- to achieve a 30% increase in the proportion of the population aged 15 and over who engage in an accumulated 30 minutes of light physical exercise most days of the week by the year 2000

- to achieve a 20% increase in the proportion of the population aged 15 and over who engage in moderate exercise for at least 20 minutes, three times a week, by the year 2000.

The Chief Executive Officers of the Health Boards, as a response to the Health Strategy targets on exercise, have established – through the Office for Health Gain – a group which is currently drawing up a strategy for the promotion of physical exercise in Ireland. The main focus of the strategy will be to increase moderate activity in the population as a whole. However, each Health Board may need to identify priority groups depending on local needs.

Progress: The promotion of physical activity has not traditionally been a mainstream activity for health professionals. If the Health Strategy targets are to be achieved, it will be necessary for the health service to give a lead and to involve other agencies, e.g. local authorities who provide their recreational facilities, the Department of Education (particularly its Sports Strategy Section), and other groups. Given that some countries such as the UK have just started in a serious way to promote exercise among their populations, it is difficult to say how successful we will be in increasing exercise levels among the Irish population.

Blood pressure

High blood pressure is one of the major risk factors for coronary heart disease, and also puts people at risk for stroke and kidney disease. Many people who have high blood pressure are not aware of the fact because they do not have any symptoms. The population target set in the Health Promotion Strategy is that 75% of the population will have a normal blood pressure level by the year 2000. As blood pressure measurement is a relatively simple examination to carry out, it is recommended that general practitioners should do this on an opportunistic basis.

Progress: Data currently available on the prevalence of detected and undetected high blood pressure are not as good as one would like. However, we do know that many cases of high blood pressure are not detected or not treated adequately. Progress over the next ten years or so will depend greatly on the extent to which we can detect and treat high blood pressure.

Inequalities in health

One of the most obvious inequalities in health status in most countries is that between men and women. For example, men have higher overall death rates than women at all ages. Some of this inequality is probably biological, but much of it is due to lifestyle and, in particular, to risk-taking behaviour. Men have higher death rates from cardiovascular disease in the middle-aged group, and have higher death rates from certain cancers like lung cancers and cancers of the bowel, and these undoubtedly contribute to differences in life expectancy. Men also have higher death rates from accidents of all kinds and suicide. The evidence is that some of this discrepancy could be bridged by behaviour modification, but it is likely that some difference will persist.

There is now an extensive research literature on variations in health. The Black Report, which commented on the unequal pattern of Britain's regional mortality, stimulated considerable interest among the public in the UK and world-wide. It has been clearly shown in the UK that there are social class gradients in mortality and that these have persisted for decades (Phillimore *et al.*, 1994; Marang-van de Mheen *et al.*, 1998). Social class gradients have been shown in relation to overall mortality, infant mortality and other health status indicators in the United States and in many other countries.

Data are scarce on how health status in Ireland varies according to socio-economic group, but there are indications that income is an important variable affecting health, with lower socio-economic status and unemployment being associated with higher mortality, morbidity and psychological stress. Some examples are listed below.

- Peri-natal mortality is highest among children of unemployed men.
- The percentage of children breast-fed (the desirable method from a health perspective) varied in 1991 from 65% among higher professional groups to 10% in the unskilled manual groups.
- Rates of admission to psychiatric hospitals are much higher in the unskilled manual group than in other socio-economic groups.
- In 1990, an Eastern Health Board study showed that standardised mortality rates were significantly higher than average in certain wards (small geographical areas with a population range from 200 to 10,000) in Dublin. These wards were areas which would be

easily recognisable as low socio-economic areas. Further studies showed that healthy lifestyles were significantly more common in the low-mortality areas than in the high-mortality areas. A subsequent study showed that lifestyle was not the only explanation for the difference in mortality rates, and that socio-economic factors have an important role.

- The Travellers' Health Status Health Study in 1987 found that life expectancy at birth is 10 years less for male travellers than for settled males, and 12 years less for women travellers than for settled women. Travellers were found to have high mortality rates, particularly from accidents and metabolic and congenital problems and also from other major causes of death.

Equity is one of the three important principles underlying the Health Strategy document, and is the value which runs through the document. The notion of equity that is most emphasised in the Health Strategy is the achievement of an equitable health service, in particular the issue of access to healthcare. Special Health Promotion interventions are, however, recommended for travellers and for those living in low socio-economic areas. The Community Mothers Project, which commenced in the Eastern Health Board in the 1980s, has been extended and is being implemented in other Health Board areas. A successful nutrition project aimed at low socio-economic groups has also been piloted in the Eastern Health Board area, and there are many other health promotion projects aimed at improving the health of those in the lower income groups.

Targeting of effective healthcare promotion and services at groups with the greatest health needs has been shown to be effective, but the impact which the health services can have on the question of equity is limited. A better distribution of economic resources would probably be the most effective means of reducing inequalities in health, and for this reason the health sector should probably be more vocal in advocating stronger social policies which would achieve this redistribution.

Health status indicators – what more is needed?

Death rates

If the achievement of health and social gain are to be the standards by which our health services will be judged, it is very important that we know how far we have progressed on the road to health gain. For this reason, we need baseline indicators which can be monitored over time. Reference has already been made to the need for health information at DED level as part of the public health common data set. In the future, it is hoped that these data will be available at DED level. In order to achieve this, a lot of work will have to be done in order to generate a computerised system for coding addresses according to DED. Relatively little work has been done in this country on the analysis of death rates by social class or by occupation. This is an important deficit given that equity in health is one of the three important principles of the Health Strategy.

Morbidity data

Specific disease registers, notification systems for communicable diseases and general practice surveillance systems are all useful methods of gathering information on morbidity in the community. The usefulness of registers has been alluded to earlier in the chapter. Other registers which would significantly contribute to our knowledge of health status in Ireland include a register of stroke, a register of coronary heart disease, a register of diabetes and a register of physical disability. There are few sentinel practice surveillance systems in Ireland for the purpose of gathering information on illnesses presenting to general practitioners. The development of such systems would be very useful in planning primary care and other services.

Lifestyle and self-perceived health

One of the major deficits in our information on health status in Ireland today is the lack of data on certain aspects of lifestyle. There is a need for a national survey which would involve samples large enough to give robust information for each Health Board on important lifestyle risk factors. This survey could include self-perceived health and might also include data from subsamples on certain physical parameters, e.g. blood cholesterol levels and body mass index. A major survey such as this might be conducted every five years. Smaller surveys giving more detail in certain areas, e.g. smoking prevalence among young people, might be conducted in the interim period to complement the major survey data.

Conclusion

The health status of a population is usually measured in terms of longevity, rates of death and illness in the population, the prevalence of illnesses, the prevalence of good and poor health practices and self-perceived health. In this country we have suffered from a lack of basic data on the health of the population. For example, no accurate baseline data are available in some areas where targets have been set in the Health Strategy. This means that we are unable to monitor progress towards these targets. It also means that we cannot be sure how realistic the targets are. Securing agreement on the more important baseline health indicators to be used for the purpose of monitoring health should be an important element of a strategy for health and social gain. These indicators should of course be consistent with the Health Strategy targets.

We are now just beginning to acquire the first elements of an Irish public health common data set, which will allow us to monitor progress towards the Health Strategy targets. However, as we are now halfway through the period set for the achievement of some of the targets, we need to consider a much greater investment in health information as a priority, in order to get a more complete picture of health patterns and trends in our population. As many of the Health Strategy targets relate to lifestyle, one of the more important priorities should be a national study on lifestyles.

Progress towards the targets can be achieved by four main strategies: better treatment of the major causes of premature deaths, improving people's lifestyles, improved co-operation between all the agencies which are in a position to influence people's health, and the adoption of public policies which promote health. Managers have a crucial role in reorienting the health services towards these strategies. The health status of the Irish population is today at an all-time high. If we follow the strategies outlined above we can expect continued progress well into the twenty-first century.

PART TWO

Direction and Control

CHAPTER 3

Irish Healthcare Policy: Legislative Strategy or Administrative Control?

David McKevitt

Introduction

Healthcare strategy in Ireland can be discussed at a number of levels. First, we can examine the legislative basis for Irish healthcare, the Health Act 1970, and enquire as to the principles or strategy underlying healthcare provision. Second, we can examine the trend of expenditure as between the different healthcare sectors – primary, community and tertiary – to see if the pattern of expenditures shows significant shifts in line with often stated policies of reorienting health policy and expenditure away from the general hospital (tertiary) sector. Third, we can examine the proposals set out in *Shaping a Healthier Future* (1994) to see if the proposed new strategy is feasible, suitable and acceptable to the many stakeholders in the system. In all our enquiries we adopt a comparative focus, to consider other countries' experience so that the Irish proposals for change can be evaluated against recent international experience.

In examining healthcare strategy, we need to see how such strategy impacts on the organisation that actually delivers the services, e.g. the hospital, community care office, child welfare clinic. This focus on the organisation is of prime importance, as much of what is written on healthcare policy is not grounded in the real world of service delivery in a context of limited resources and conflicting service priorities.

This chapter establishes this important strategy–services linkage through a model of the organisation (we call it the street-level public organisation) which takes account of and explains the environmental influences that impact on service delivery. Those influences include legislation, organisation structures and performance measurement:

they also include professional associations and associated codes of ethics and the activities of related service organisations. Strategy is concerned with the activities of service management, making explicit choices (including decisions *not* to do certain things), sustaining a long-term commitment and maintaining relationships (with clients, providers, government) in a complex environment. We will see that in Ireland the street-level public organisation delivering health services is burdened by poor performance measurement systems, inadequate professional supervision and underdeveloped management capability. Underlying this organisational context is the strategic framework for delivery of health services.

Ireland lacks a healthcare strategy that is defined and set out in legislation. No proposals exist at present to remedy this strategic deficit. This marks Ireland out as different from countries as diverse as New Zealand, Sweden and the Netherlands, and promotes the proposition that we, as a small country, can make our way in a complex social and economic environment without the benefit of other countries' experience.

The Health (Amendment) Act 1996 and the Public Service Management Act 1997 represent some changes in the framework of accountability for health services management. The Health Act 1996 clarifies the respective roles of members of Health Boards and Chief Executive Officers, seeks to improve financial accountability and obliges Health Boards to produce an annual service plan. The Bill also reduces the operational control of the Minister for Health over Health Board decisions while obliging the Health Boards to secure 'the most beneficial, effective and efficient use of resources' (Section 2). The Public Service Management (PSM) Act 1997, while not directly applicable to Health Boards, seeks to improve the management structure, systems and ethos of the central civil service through publication and Dail review of departmental strategy statements, greater flexibility in human resource management and the assignment of specific legislative duties to the Secretary-General (formerly Secretary) of departments. The PSM Act forms part of the government's Strategic Management Initiative and the wider proposals contained in *Delivering Better Government* (1996) on public service reform. It is far too early to say how these legislative proposals will work in practice: indeed, there is an urgent need for evaluative studies of their impact to assess their effect on service delivery. For this chapter's purpose we can acknowledge the trend towards greater accountability, improved management structures and greater financial accountability. This represents an advance in the framework of control, but still leaves open the more important question – what is the strategic intent of Irish healthcare policy, and how does Ireland's strategy stand up to comparison with that of other modern economies?

Almost ten years ago, in a comparative study of healthcare strategy across a number of European countries, this author (McKevitt, 1989) observed that:

> A central stance of the findings is that control in healthcare yields similar challenges to politicians, civil servants, and healthcare professionals under different financial systems for health service delivery... Control, *per se*, is rectificatory and not restorative; that is, it is about the maintenance of norms, the following of patterns and rules once these have been laid down. *In Ireland, control was not seen in this way, largely because the legislative framework did not contain any explicit strategy.* Decisions on resource allocations were not related to any specific objectives, nor was the performance of healthcare professionals subject to any sustained scrutiny.

As we shall see later in this chapter, very little has changed since this observation was made. Legislative proposals are set out in *Shaping a Healthier Future*, but are primarily organisational and structural and do not address the strategic deficit at the centre of Irish healthcare policy: the absence of specific and measurable strategy objectives that guide the resource allocation process, subject professionals and management to appropriate performance measurement and give the citizen a voice in the service delivery process.

This chapter is based on the following arguments.

- To be effective, healthcare policy has to be set out in legislation, as it is in other countries, and the activities of professionals and managers measured and controlled.
- The street-level public organisations (SLPOs) delivering health services are subject to conflicting environmental forces, and public-sector managers have to manage these conflicts in a consensual way
- Healthcare policy is emergent and incremental, and policy development is not the responsibility solely of the Department of Health.

Healthcare strategy and legislation

The following principles underlying proposed legislative change are set out in Chapter 3 of *Shaping a Healthier Future*.

- The Minister and Department should be responsible for the development of health policy and overall control of expenditure, but should not be involved in the detailed management of the health services.
- Greater responsibility should be devolved to the appropriate executive agencies.
- The roles of all key parties, including the boards and management of the statutory authorities, must be clearly defined.
- Greater autonomy must be balanced by increased accountability at all levels, and there must be independent monitoring and evaluation of the performance of the executive agencies.

In a very important qualifier, the document goes on to state that 'the legislation will be general in nature and will provide a framework within which the statutory and voluntary agencies will operate'. We have seen that some of these changes are provided for in the Health (Amendment) Act 1996.

In strategic terms, the proposals set out above constitute some progress on the Health Act 1970, yet their primary aim and purpose remain organisational and structural. One important example will illustrate this strategic deficit – *Shaping a Healthier Future* is replete with references to the equity considerations that are said to underlie healthcare policy, yet nowhere in the principles underlying the legislation does equity or equality of resource usage merit an inclusion. *Shaping a Healthier Future* also emphasises accountability, performance measurement, monitoring of service levels, etc., yet, again, nowhere is there a strategic objective (set out in the proposed legislation) against which this monitoring will take place. How then can progress towards achievement of strategy be measured?

In this context, we can note that Swedish legislation (June 1985, Act HS-90) sets out what healthcare on equal terms requires: '(a) equality in the supply of resources available throughout different parts of the country; (b) equality in the utilisation of care between different groups in society; (c) equality in terms of access to care; (d) equality in terms of quality and efficiency of care'. In this example, there is a clear legislative balance between strategy, measurement and management. A general statement of legislative strategy (*note:* not policy, which in any event it is not proposed to include in the Irish legislation) provides a framework for evaluation, a means through which performance can be evaluated and a benchmark from which future resource allocations can be measured. It is true that Swedish healthcare policy, like other areas of its welfare provision, has been the subject of reform in the 1990s. Such reforms, largely based on changes in county council control frameworks, have stressed economic efficiency rather than equity considerations. However, the primary importance of legislation remains: Sweden has a legislative statement of healthcare strategy and its performance measurement framework is oriented towards evaluation of these strategic objectives. Therefore, we can speak of strategy in Swedish healthcare provision, assess its effectiveness and evaluate its performance. We cannot have a similar debate in Ireland due to the absence of a legislative expression of healthcare strategy.

The New Zealand Health and Disability Services Act 1993 defined the reform of public provision and funding of health and disability services as being to secure for the people of New Zealand

- the best health
- the best care or support for those in need of such services
- the greatest independence for people with disabilities

that is reasonably achievable within the amount of funding provided.

A National Advisory Committee on Core Health and Disability Support Services was appointed in 1992 to advise the Government on the fairest and most effective use of public monies for such services. In its first two reports, the Committee recognised that public priorities that should be emphasised are as follows:

- mental health and substance abuse
- children's health services
- integrated community care services
- emergency ambulance services
- habilitation and rehabilitation services
- hospice services.

The Committee also identified in its first report 'considerable unfairness in the access people have to services in different parts of the country'. The work of the Committee is based on extensive public consultation, discussion documents, working with medical providers and drafting ethical guidelines on the principles that should be used to define care services and 'to guide decisions about the allocation of resources to core health and disability services'.

The Committee, in its report for 1994–95, recommended that the Regional Health Authorities give increasing emphasis to the service priorities outlined above.

Central to the New Zealand health reforms was the contractor–provider arrangement, whereby Regional Authorities would purchase, under contract, a service from Crown health enterprises – primarily, but not exclusively, hospitals. The responsibility of the Minister for Health was restricted to monitoring the performance of the health system. In this regard, the New Zealand reforms (which are still far from completion) go well beyond those prefigured in the Irish proposals, as Regional Authorities are concerned with promotion of health objectives and not with the actual provision of services. As such they form part of a wider civil and public service reform (McKevitt, 1996) that is driven by a series of legislation (see Table 3.1). We can see that in the New Zealand case, legislation of a strategic nature was the primary instrument of reform. It could be argued that a single model of reform, applied across all sectors, including the commercial state sector, is inappropriate: that healthcare is not the same as education, for example; that the purchaser contract model ignores, or does not take account of, important human aspects of the service delivery. What is relevant to Ireland is the specificity of legislation, the concentration on measurement of performance and the widespread use of information databases to track achievement.

It is also the case that in New Zealand's healthcare policy a 'community of interests' was not acknowledged and reforms were based solely on the market model (McKevitt, 1998). This is something which many might not find appropriate in an Irish context. Yet it is also the case that in Ireland we have a 'mixed provision' of public and private care which is totally facilitated through the activities of healthcare professionals – hospital consultants – who are themselves public employees. The undermanagement of the service plans provisions of the Common Contract allows for the unregulated practice of private provision utilising public facilities. There is clearly, therefore, an important issue of management control in the street-level public organisation delivering health services. This lack of control is strategic rather than operational: that is, it will not be resolved

Table 3.1. New Zealand administrative and legislative reforms (McKevitt, 1996)

1986 State Owned Enterprises Act

Separates commercial activities from government departments; commercial criteria provide an assessment of managerial performance; board members are appointed primarily from the private sector.

1988 State Sector Act

Personnel and industrial relations for civil servants are placed on a par with private-sector arrangements; increased accountability is assigned to senior managers. The Act explicitly assumes that employers, unions, and workers in the state and private sectors are treated in the same way unless there is a compelling case for different treatment.

1989 State Sector Amendment Act

Extends the principle of management and accountability contained in the State Sector Act into the education service; the amendment confers normal employer rights to employers in the education service, places senior positions in secondary schools on contract, and provides for national criteria for assessing teacher performance.

1989 Public Finance Act

Provides for new contractual relationships between heads of government departments (chief executives) and ministers. Departments are required to adopt accrual accounting, to give them more complete financial information and to enable costs of outputs to be more easily measured. Chief executives are appointed on performance-linked contracts of up to five years. The budgetary process is altered so that the two separate interests of government, as purchaser of the outputs of the department and as owner of the department's assets, are separated.

1991 Employment Contracts Act

Employees of the state have the choice of whether to belong to any form of employees' organisation (which may be a union) formed to represent their interests. Employers and employees are free to negotiate over whether to have individual or collective contracts and, subject to the Act and other legislation, their content. The number, type and mix of contracts to apply in a particular workplace are negotiable.

---

through improved accounting frameworks; rather it requires strategic change at the legislative level to separate public and private provision. Ireland has a very underdeveloped performance measurement framework for both professionals and management: lacking this essential guidance mechanism, we need hardly wonder why the street-level public organisation is subject to endemic unresolved tensions.

The striking difference between healthcare provision in Ireland and in the Netherlands is that the latter is supported primarily through private health insurance, with central government paying some 15% of healthcare expenditures. Traditionally, healthcare provision in the Netherlands has been a private-sector enterprise and government has restricted its role to one of supervision and regulation. In the hospital sector, 90% of acute beds are in non-government-controlled institutions. In 1974, the Government formulated three policy goals for the health sector: equal access to health services, even distribution of health facilities over the country, and a decline in the growth of health expenditures. The growth rate fell from 10.7% in 1977 to 7% in 1982 and 4.3% in 1983. In 1985 the growth rate was 1.5%.

In 1972 the Hospital Facilities Act was passed, which began the process of volume control in the hospitals. A licence was required from the Ministry of Health to build or extend a facility which required an investment of more than 500,000 Dutch guilders. In 1979, the Amended Hospital Facilities Act required Provincial Government to draw up regional hospital plans, and on this basis licences could be granted for constructing or reconstructing hospital facilities. The regulation of specialisms within hospitals was controlled through the Sickness Funds Insurance Act, which allowed the Funds to refuse contracts for new specialisms. The 1982 Health Services Act, which replaced the Amended Hospital Facilities Act, allowed regulation of the volume and quality of services. Since 1983, central government introduced regulations that required short-term acute hospitals to operate under a fixed budget system; the budgets were set at each institution's expenditure level of two years prior, adjusted for subsequent inflation. Hospitals which borrow funds on the capital markets used to have a State guarantee for these borrowings, but this was ended in 1987.

The Netherlands provides a striking contrast, in terms of its system of control, to the Irish experience. Yet, unlike Ireland, the Netherlands has primarily a private (or, more accurately, a corporatist) healthcare sector in terms of organisation and finance. The impetus for state regulation resides in the Dutch tradition since the 1960s of increasing state involvement in social services provision, and income maintenance supports which are generally classified as 'Welfare State'. Dutt and Costa (1985), in a review of public planning in the Netherlands, describe the rationale for state involvement as follows:

> Where care changes from being a favour to a right guaranteed by government, it is natural that government should take the initiative in planning and harmonisation... in the first place, the initiative for planning legislation developed partly in order to meet the wish for the right to co-determination expressed by the democratising movements. Thus, there is opposition to planning legislation from private organisations and allied politicians.

The degree of regulation can also impede what professionals and consumers might regard as welcome initiatives in medical care treatment. Thus, for example, the regulatory cycle for new technology or treatment provision can take two years or more to complete and, hence, can restrict the diffusion and application of new technology.

The Netherlands has sought to constrain health expenditures and the behaviour of the providers (hospitals and doctors) through an extensive system of legislation and regulation. This has proved successful in dampening down expenditure growth, while there is evidence that consumer groups have effectively bypassed restrictions on technological application. Discretion in decision-making is very tightly constrained at a time of general unease over the growth in health service administrative costs. The 'trade-off' made in terms of control as against consumer choice (the sickness funds are private insurance funds) is not a final one. New legislation may well see a retreat from the current regulatory system to one where more choice is exercised by individuals. While disquiet has been expressed in the Netherlands over the administrative costs of the system of regulation, this is in the context of state control of the activities of private health insurance funds.

The proposals contained in *Shaping a Healthier Future* cover organisational relationships, measurement of specific healthcare targets (a very welcome development) and the clarification of responsibilities as between the boards and members of Health Authorities (formerly Health Boards). In one sense, such proposals can be seen as operational management issues, in so far as they do not touch on the strategic objectives of the system. The legislation does not itself address strategic objectives except in so far as it sees the Department of Health as having responsibility for health policy (see below). Measurement and control systems, if they are to be effective and relevant, must relate to the strategic objectives of the enterprise or organisation; feedback on performance and achievement is relevant only if overall strategy is agreed and explicit at the national level. The Swedish, Dutch and New Zealand examples all show evidence of measurement and control systems that are tied to specific legislative objectives.

One can criticise the New Zealand system for being overly prescriptive in the rigour of its contractor–provider mechanism, and the Dutch for detailed regulatory provision. The Swedish system, while very strong on monitoring of new technology and procedures, has hitherto lacked clear governance of its healthcare professionals.

To critique international comparisons is valid; it means that as a country, Ireland can learn from them. Yet in Ireland's case we have proposed a legislative framework that is silent on strategy, and a relationship with providers that is positively hands-off in terms of measurement of effectiveness. It may well be that, as a country, we do not wish to be explicit as to the principles which underlie our healthcare strategy and do not wish to incorporate such principles in legislation. We must, however, recognise that measurement and accountability then become a mechanical and routinised activity – the operational drives out the strategic. Similarly, performance of professionals (and, indeed, managers) becomes problematic: what benchmarks or standards do we apply to measure strategic success?

Street-level public organisations

As stated above, health service organisations, like many public-sector organisations, are subject to conflicting environmental challenges and economic, professional, judicial and competing-resource priorities. Professional bureaucracies such as hospitals are complex organisations, difficult to manage, and the location for energetic debate and conflict on service priorities. The health service organisation also has to respond to (or at least be seen to take notice of) citizen demands for service improvements, the political pressures for accountability and efficiency and professional claims for resource additions to sustain new service developments. It is at the point of the SLPO that strategy and service management meet: in the absence of planned and co-ordinated strategy, the SLPO becomes subject to conflicting demands. How can the public-sector manager decide between conflicting priorities in a way that is defensible and legitimate?

The first step in this process of accountability is to understand the environment within which the SLPO operates: such understanding includes both the *outer* context (the law, professional practices) and the *inner* context (service priorities, organisation structure) of the SLPO. If this management context is understood, we will be better able to relate and improve strategy and operational management of service delivery.

How are we to make sense of the endemic tensions within public organisations in the general area of social welfare, including health-care? Such tensions are exemplified by uneasy relations between central government on the one hand and professionals in SLPOs as well as the professional bodies themselves on the other.

To see the source of the problem, we need to construct a model of the specific influences from the environment that play on service delivery of public organisations. For our purpose, we adapt the Open Systems Model of Organisations, originally developed by Bruce Scott (1962) at the Harvard Business School, because this particular model highlights the workings of subunits (part/whole relationships), and contains the notion – important for our purpose – that each subunit is best understood as responding to the various forces in its own particular environment. In the words of Scott:

> Briefly, our model asserts that (1) any organisation relates to its environment via a strategy for advancing its interests as it perceives those interests; (2) the interests of the various subunits of an organisation often differ from those of the organisation as a whole; and (3) thus the central or general headquarters of the organisation must bring continuous influence to bear on the subunits in order to motivate them to act in conformity, not with their own divergent interests, but with the general or shared interest of the organisation as a whole.

Scott goes on to highlight the forms of influence available:

> Among the various modes of influence which the headquarters has at its disposal, four are of particular importance – the ability (1) to allocate

53

resources; (2) to establish and alter organisational structures; (3) to measure and reward individuals and subunits; (4) to formulate policy limits or rules of the game.

We would expand this model and add a fifth feature, general legislation, which is a key feature of the public sector. Fig. 3.1 outlines the general model of the street-level organisation in its environment.

Using this model and noting from the data gathered in my field research in the UK, Sweden, New Zealand and Germany that service delivery in the area of social welfare is a managed process, we can move now to examine the essence of the management task involved, i.e. relating a street-level public organisation to its environment. The question then is what are the key points in the environment itself. It is in this respect that data from field research, over a period of time in a number of countries, are vital. Fig. 3.2 represents my research finding of the recurring tension points in the environment of SLPOs.

It will be noted that the immediate source of recurring tensions is point A, the relations between central government and the professions. The model enables us to see an essential fact: SLPOs are under a dual set of influences. From central government there are four modes of influence (general legislation, allocation of resources, organisational structure, and performance measurement), each of which is powerful, and the four together are extremely powerful.

Without established, accepted and enforced rules of the game, as is known from research on private enterprise, the effect of these four powerful modes of influence can cause the activities of SLPOs to run wild and undirected. Because each of these four modes of influence plays mainly on individual self-interest, it is the rules of the game – the ethical codes – that are needed to harness the forces of self-interest to social goals. Rules of the game really are important, and of paramount importance is the fact that these rules are established by a quite different kind of institution, namely the professions. If there is a solid relationship between government and the professions, the inevitable tensions at point A can be resolved without adverse impact on the SLPO. If the relationship is poor, then the tension at point A will debilitate the whole system of service delivery, as my research in the UK makes quite clear. In the social welfare area of the public sector, good relations between government and the professions are important for success in quality service delivery.

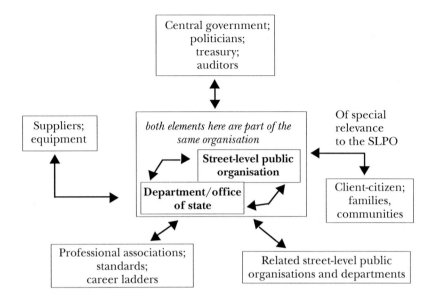

Source: McKevitt (1996).

Fig. 3.1. Model of the SLPO, the department/office of state and their environment

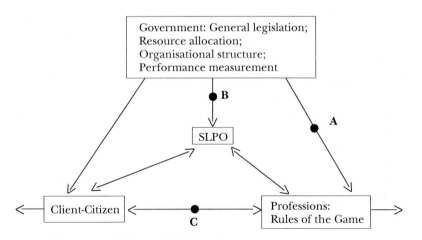

Source: Wrigley and McKevitt (1995), p. 24.

Fig. 3.2. Conflicting environmental forces

In the Irish context, government–professional relations mainly centre on remuneration – there is little, if any, sustained dialogue on performance in service delivery. Certainly there is no scrutiny of client satisfaction with professional service delivery, nor any independent scrutiny like that of the Health Ombudsman in Britain. The relationship is a distant one and is not conducive to easy management in the street level organisation.

However, government influence on SLPOs may be fundamentally impaired by problems in general legislation as at point B in Fig. 3.2. McKevitt (1989) in his study of healthcare policy in Ireland, used a comparative approach whereby, in certain crucial aspects, Ireland was compared with other modern countries, including Sweden and Holland. McKevitt then explained that:

> The Swedish and Dutch systems, in contrast to Ireland, share common features in their concern for explicitness in legislation, their attendance to the sovereign importance of measurement and control systems, and their willingness to adapt and modify their control system to refocus their investment decisions.

From this view, we can see that any defect in the legislative framework which impairs the process of resource allocation will lead to recurring fundamental tensions between central government and professional associations in the environment of SLPOs.

In public service delivery and investment decisions, legislation is pivotal to any strategy that requires a change in the pattern of resource allocation to underpin new policies. Most public service managers instinctively understand the inertial force of a pattern of incremental resource allocation; this year's increment (or decrement) of resources is justified on the basis of last year's allocation. The legislation we evaluated confirms this proposition: the pattern of investment in social provision, reflecting as it does consensus and compromise among many stakeholders, is built up over considerable periods of time. If countries wish to change these patterns then legislation is required to shift the balance of investment allocation: treasury officials are unmoved by policy objectives without the backing of legislation. In parliamentary democracies, legislation gives legitimacy and status to policy objectives and captures the high ground in policy decisions in investment priorities.

An instructive example of how legislation and investment

decisions can be a source of management challenge is the Child Care Act 1991. A comprehensive statement of policy in this important area, which lays very specific and extensive obligations on the Health Boards, was not accompanied by appropriate strategic investment. Or, more accurately, the additional investment monies made available to underpin child-care services were allocated in an environment where competing professional interests were vying for the investment – medical, management, nursing, social worker.

The Health Boards struggle to develop appropriate and feasible strategies in a context of disputed priorities, inadequate control and underdeveloped management practice. The specificity of the Child Care Act also increases the legal contestability of Health Board performance: while such contestability is to be welcomed, it does place additional responsibilities on managers in a multi-professional organisation. The working out of appropriate strategies in this area may well provide a benchmark for management practice in other service areas. Clearly, one criterion for organisational success is partner-ship and commitment of professional providers to a common organisational objective.

We can reflect that the absence of a legislative strategy to under-pin some of the major UK policy shifts in education and healthcare probably accounts for their relative lack of success. We do not, of course, propose the view that legislation, even if it is cast in a strategic dimension such as found in Swedish healthcare, is a guarantee of strategic control. Policy-makers have numerous and conflicting demands on their attention, and legislation can also be viewed as partly a symbolic act, which represents good intentions rather than administrative clarity.

Our research indicates that another fundamental source of the tension may well lie at point C in Fig. 3.2 above, namely a break in the natural relationship between the community of citizens and the professional bodies.

In English-speaking countries at least, where the prevailing culture may feature individualism, the professions can and sometimes do in their practices go too far ahead of social sentiment, thereby essentially becoming isolated bodies in the environment. Govern-ments cannot do this because of the democratic system. Thus, in the English-speaking countries, the rules of the game, the code of professional ethics, may evolve in ways that go too far outside the boundaries provided by social sentiment, and therefore be a funda-mental source of tension in the environment between client-citizens and the professions. The most conspicuous example in the early 1990s of such tension in the United Kingdom was provided by the system of primary education.

There need not be any inherent conflict between professional ethics and mainstream management requirements for an efficient and accountable service. Historically, the medical and social service professions have been granted a large degree of autonomy on matters of discipline, standards of service and internal control. Indeed, the market model of service provision seeks to challenge professional independence directly, through specification of contracts for service delivery and related performance measurement frameworks. A contract is, however, a blunt and costly instrument (witness the multi-million pound administrative expenditure in the UK on the main-tenance of the 'internal market'), and does not provide sufficiently for citizen 'voice' in the appraisal of service quality. A more pragmatic and feasible model is that of partnership and consensus between professionals and management found in Scandinavian and other northern European countries; here professional 'freedom' is legitimated and controlled through democratic partnership and social obligation. Such control also takes place, as we have seen, in a context of specific strategic objectives set out in legislation. A form of 'new managerialism' is evident in the PSM Act 1997, whereby managerial accountability is seen as the 'best way' to provide services. It is apparent that other successful countries combine management with profes-sional co-operation. It is to be hoped that Ireland will not adopt a managerial ethos that precludes professional 'voice': such a strategy has clearly failed in the UK.

An additional source of tension is the absence of any sustained or systematic appraisal of professional performance within the system. The contracts for general practitioners and hospital consultants are primarily contracts of employment, without any structured monitoring of performance. In incentive terms, GPs now have less motivation to see medical card patients, thus placing additional pressures on self-referral to hospital accident and emergency departments. Hospital consultants, through their unregulated access to hospital resources for private patients, have incentives to allocate more time to private practice. There is no budgetary control system which allows for transparency in the formal separation of costs for public and private users of hospital care. Designing information systems in hospitals will yield useful information; without attending to the larger issue of incentive structures, the conflict of interests will remain. Here we can see how the tension points at A and B in Fig. 3.2 are interrelated: the absence of strategic objectives in legislation fetters the usefulness of any performance measurement system for professionals, and hence further reduces the likelihood of achieving any consensual arrangement for joint monitoring of strategic implementation of health policy.

There is, therefore, a dual weakness in the Irish framework of strategic control: first, legislation which does not provide strategic objectives against which resource allocation and goal achievement can be assessed; and second, inadequate monitoring of professional activity against appropriate policy objectives. This lack of strategic control matters greatly to the SLPO; without a clear linkage between strategic objectives (at national level) and the operational management of the organisation (at regional level), managing is simply an exercise in resource management unconnected with any overall strategy. If strategy is not set out in legislative terms, the 'rules of the game' and other means of influence open to managers (rewards and punishments, organisational structures) become zero-sum games, where one department's gain is another department's loss.

Clearly, at the level of health sectors (primary, community and tertiary), resource allocation will not shift appreciably in the absence of legislative strategy; the inertia of incremental budgeting will ensure the primacy of the hospital sector. New Zealand, as we have seen, probably overemphasises the monitoring of provider performance (to the detriment of equity considerations), while the UK model of micro-efficiency ignores the strategic unity of the system. Ireland, on the other hand, ignores both strategic specificity *and* the 'rules of the game', both essential features of strategic control.

Health policy and strategy process

The legislative proposals set out in *Shaping a Healthier Future* include the principle that:

> The Minister and Department shall be responsible for the development of health policy and overall control of expenditure but should not be involved in the detailed management of the service.

Such a policy prescription is based on the idea that policy and implementation are two separate processes: the centre sets the policy, the agencies execute it. Such a prescription is not consistent with much recent strategy research, whereby it is seen that there is a continuous and iterative cycle between policy and implementation. In strategic terms, the policy prescription can be described as a deliberate strategy. In the general strategy field, for a *deliberate* strategy to be realised, the following conditions have to be satisfied:

- precise intentions must exist in the organisation, so that there can be no doubt about what was desired *prior to* any action being taken
- such intentions have to be shared by virtually all actors, either because they accept them or in response to controls
- the intentions must be realised exactly as intended.

The environment must therefore be benign, predictable and controllable. Clearly, the healthcare environment, which is characterised by complex social, technical, economic and ethical forces, does not allow for such conditions to be satisfied. Nor in the proposed deliberate strategy can the compliance of individual actors (manager, professionals and clients) be assured – especially in the case of professionals whose performance is not subject to any structured review.

An emergent or consensus strategy, on the other hand, reflecting as it does the convergence of patterns of behaviour based on mutual adjustment, grows out of adaptation and learning from the environment. The strategy evolves without centrally defined prior intentions, and it is driven by collective action. Such a strategy more accurately reflects the complex world of SLPOs, subject as they are to conflicting environmental forces. It is also more consistent with the complex trade-offs and mutual adjustment that exist in the healthcare environment. Emergence does not preclude senior management (or Department of Health) involvement; their role, though, is one of facilitation and support rather than a reliance on policy directives. Indeed, the recently established Office for Health Gain is a good example of such facilitation and support.

Legislation embodying strategic objectives provides an 'umbrella' strategy which can guide and direct the system. Emergence and consensus can be facilitated by such legislation and the activities of the SLPO controlled, albeit with more explicit attendance to performance measurement. Policy statements are no substitute for legislative strategy. Policy can, in any event, be subverted or ignored by both professionals and managers in the SLPO, not through acts of defiance but simply through the adaptation of their collective actions to the environmental conditions they face.

The idea that policy legitimately resides solely at the strategic apex of the organisation is outmoded and does not reflect the complex professional world of healthcare organisations. Organisational restructuring and performance assessment *logically* follow from a change in strategy. Such a strategic change requires legislative expression incorporating specific and measurable objectives. Without attending to this important strategic issue, Ireland will continue to impose mechanical control in a complex environment. Compliance of professionals and managers cannot be assumed; it has to be given direction and support through appropriate legislation and the adoption of strategic processes appropriate to the SLPO.

Conclusion

What can we conclude from this review of Irish healthcare strategy, and especially its legislative underpinning as outlined in *Shaping a Healthier Future?* This chapter has taken a very specific focus, applying the experience of other countries to Ireland, especially in the field of legislation. It has also presented a model for looking at the street-level public organisations (SLPOs) where the actual work of service delivery takes place. It has been argued that strategy should be seen as consensual and emergent, and less dependent on policy.

Strategic legislative objectives and mutual co-operation and adjustment are supportive of professional service organisations. A legislative strategy would be *suitable* to the healthcare environment; it would most certainly address the issues of equity of access and geographic distribution of resources. It would place Ireland on a par with other developed nations.

How *feasible* would such a strategy be? Here we must look at both the national and regional levels. At national level, an explicit strategy would guide and direct resource allocation (in strategic terms a 10 year period would be appropriate) towards different sectoral levels of the system, and it would incorporate a measurement and control function linked to specific objectives. At regional level, where the SLPOs operate, a policy of emergent consensus has to operate to fit local circumstances and the professional base of the service. However, the SLPO needs assistance from the centre in the installation of appropriate performance measurement system for professionals – such systems do not need to be mechanistic; they can be structured to tie in with the professional ethics of service delivery.

Equally, managers will need training and development in the management of the SLPO; such management needs to take account of the environmental forces operating on the SLPO, in particular 'citizen voice'. It is obvious that this aspect of SLPO life will become more dominant in the years ahead.

The recent publication of a Charter for Customer Service for Government Departments as part of *Delivering Better Government* (1997), together with the NESF (1995) report *Quality Delivery of Social Services*, points to the increasing prominence being given to the idea of customer service. How realistic it is to view such initiatives as significant, it is too early to say. A major study of UK experience (McKevitt & Lawton, 1996) found that public organisations gave increased attention to performance indicators that stressed institutional and managerial functions to the detriment of citizen voice. Indeed, the study also found evidence for a tentative alliance between professionals and citizens in their resistance to resource cutbacks that impacted on service delivery. In Ireland we are a long way from a performance framework that would measure professional activity, let alone one that would promote citizen voice. Yet if managers are to manage the environment of the SLPO strategically, they will need to give attention to this important part of the organisation. An increasing awareness of citizen voice, together with the regulatory powers of the courts, means that the procedural integrity of management decisions is more open to scrutiny.

How *acceptable* will the proposals outlined be to the stakeholders in the system? It is quite likely that the Department or, more relevantly, the Minister will be resistant to the argument for a legislative strategy, seeing it as fettering their discretion or room for manoeuvre. Such a reaction is understandable, if misplaced. All relevant international examples point to the need for a legislative statement of strategy; it can be fashioned to suit specific Irish circumstances, but there is no doubt that it is required.

Professionals may resist what they perceive as measurement systems that impinge on their freedom of operation; world-wide the trend is towards consensual management of SLPOs, and incentives can be built in to ease the necessary transition. The managers will have a more specific set of objectives and the freedom to evolve appropriate policy initiatives within the umbrella of corporate strategy. The citizen-client can look to a more accountable system built, not on the exigencies of budgets, but on the clear requirements of the law.

CHAPTER 4

Governance – Where the Dream Starts and the Buck Stops

SEAN CONROY

Introduction

Disputes, scandals and dysfunction in government, semi-state, sporting, healthcare and business organisations in the past decade, and most noticeably in the past few years, have often shared one conspicuous feature: confused governance. Either faulty governance processes have resulted in problems or problems have been unresolved because of faulty governance processes. Despite the myriad boards in existence, these faults have resulted in the buck whizzing past boards and either stopping only when it has reached the office of Minister or Taoiseach or, worse, not stopping anywhere.

The problem is not unique to Ireland. Board members in North America have been described as 'the well-intentioned in relentless pursuit of the trivial'. Where the requirement and opportunity for leadership are greatest, the job description and performance are weakest.

Before developing further what appears so far to be a bleak assessment, I pause here to assert that governance can be redesigned and that any organisation that undertakes this challenge will be enriched and will effect its desired outcomes in the greater society of which it is a part.

What goes wrong in the process of governance? Why do so many Board Members and Chief Executive Officers/Presidents/Directors find it so frustrating and yet feel so helpless? What would we expect of well-functioning governance? How can we get there?

Governance – what is it?

Governance is authoritative strategic leadership by a group of people exercising the ownership of an organisation. Put another way, governance is the exercise of ownership. Another way again: govern-ance is the extreme end of management, exercised by a group of individuals acting as one. One last shot: governance is where the dreams start and the buck stops.

The writer's background is teacher, then engineer, then doctor, now manager-doctor. Eleven years in Canada included clinical and managerial appointments as well as work with the Canadian Council for Health Services Accreditation as a hospital surveyor. During the 1990s in Canada, dramatic restructuring of healthcare began. Hospitals closed; others merged. Issues of ownership and governance came to the fore. The writer was involved in this restructuring process and became interested in ownership. The focus of this chapter is healthcare governance.

Boards are exceeded in authority only by owners; they act in trust for these owners (for example, in healthcare, the Minister, a Religious Order, a Society). The essential role given in trust is the ownership role. Thus governance is firstly the exercise of ownership. Another unique feature of boards is that governance is vested in a group of people, rather than an individual. In healthcare, there is an example of an even more interesting challenge: Health Boards meet in the presence of the media and act in trust for an owner (the Minister), not entirely clear as to how much ownership he has devolved to them.

Problems in governance

Flaws in governance are common to all organisations in society. Operational details infest board agendas. Boards follow staff rather than lead them; many would suffer paralysis if required to compile their own agendas. Crisis management blocks policy formulation. Monitoring of staff activity substitutes for stipulating desired outcomes. Executive/Board relationships are ill-defined and issues in this area, when they arise, are solved on an *ad hoc* basis rather than recognised as powerful opportunities to clarify roles. In part, Health Boards function poorly because the owner is too involved. In part, the owner is too involved because Health Boards function poorly.

All boards at various times recognise that they are experiencing problems, and most make efforts at corrective action. This action is usually no more than symptom control. Boards get more involved in the organisation (multiple committees, endless meetings, agendas packed with operational matters) or less ('let the Chief Executive Officer do the job'; 'tell us what you want approved'). Boards or Board Chairmen elbow the Chief Executive Officer out of the way and assume day-to-day management or retreat into embarrassed impotence ('we're only volunteers'). Boards decide their role is communicating with staff and boosting morale, or seclude themselves in the minutiae of long-range planning. Boards become inquisitors of their Chief Executive Officer or high-profile fan clubs for their Chief Executive Officer. The same board at different junctures can adopt any of the above styles, usually as a reaction to a perceived problem of the moment. It is difficult to lead reactively. We cannot afford to continue to sentence well-meaning people to penal servitude on dysfunctional boards or to sentence organisations to governance without leadership. We can liberate boards to create the energy and vision we know to be probable when groups of individuals act with synergy. Society has long known of the moral power of such activity; we have a jury system in our courts.

A particular difficulty arises in governance as practised by Health Boards. While boards that operate well are composed of members who know that they have an ownership (and hence leadership) role – a mandate – many Health Board members come to the table seeking mandates, i.e. political election, re-election or advancement. While posturing is part of the dynamics of any board, politicians sitting on such boards in the presence of the media are particularly prone to it. This is not to say they are uninterested in or incapable of exercising good governance. In the absence of an appropriate job description and model of governance, however, who can blame them for pursuing the goal they best understand – albeit a personal, party or professional goal?

The need for some fundamental changes in healthcare is recognised, as the following quotations from *Shaping a Healthier Future* illustrate.

- Recognising that our existing organisational structures are in many ways incapable of achieving this agenda for change the Government has decided on a range of organisational reforms.
- The Minister and Department should be responsible for the development of health policy and overall control of expenditure but should not be involved in the detailed management of the health services.

- Greater responsibility should be devolved to the appropriate executive agencies.
- The roles of all key parties, including the boards and managements of the statutory authorities, must be clearly defined.
- Greater autonomy must be balanced by increased accountability at all levels and there must be independent monitoring and evaluation of the performance of the executive agencies.
- Some decisions require to be taken at national level to ensure uniform access to services and for budgetary reasons. On the other hand, operational decisions are best taken locally with local knowledge.
- The division of health administration into eight regions has worked well since its introduction in 1971 and has provided a strong element of local democracy in the health services.
- Policy functions will be carried out directly by the boards while operational functions will be delegated to management. Of course, the Chief Executive Officer and his/her management team will have a key role in the development of policy, but the board's ultimate responsibility for the decisions will be unambiguous.
- The legislation will specify that the following functions are reserved for the boards of the authorities:
    - deciding on a multi-annual strategic plan based on the identified needs of its population and taking account of statutory requirements and national policy guidelines
    - determining, at the beginning of each year, the level of services to be provided within the expenditure limits set by the allocation
    - agreeing and submitting to the Minister a budget for those services within the expenditure limits determined by the allocation.

It is not clear to the author that governance is specifically recognised as functioning poorly and in need of the radical change proposed here. On one hand, the 'Health Strategy' appears to promise that the Department of Health will devolve more ownership to Health Boards (to be known as Health Authorities); this would require a focus on governance. On the other hand, one can infer an ambivalence as to what is to be further devolved, policy formulation or policy implementation. If the intention is to devolve 'operations' primarily, Health Authority governance is not seen as a major issue; there will not be much of it. The boards of these authorities will function as Line or Advisory Boards rather that Governing Boards; they will be puppet regimes. Given the history of tight central control of healthcare, the inferred ambivalence may indeed be present in Department of Health thinking. Or perhaps there really is a vague, poorly articulated worry about the ability of Health Authority boards to govern.

Characteristics of good governance

There is none the less an opportunity for these boards now, because of the real governance they can involve themselves in if they develop the ten characteristics set out below. This opportunity exists even if 'devolution' is slow or incomplete. It will beget more devolution.

What should we expect of a successful board? What would its characteristics be? If these can be teased out, the rebirth of governance can occur. A good board will:

1. *create ideas* – if the board cannot continuously question the reasons for the organisation's existence in society, who can? Boards have to 'dream'.
2. *set the tone* – every organisation needs a set of values, a mission, from which all effort flows. These 'first principles' are constantly there for staff, markers that help them reorient when they feel off-track or lost.
3. *decide the desired results* – organisational activities are often regarded, wrongly, as results. The board must state what effect it wants its organisation to have on society, an effect, end or outcome that staff activity must produce. The means are a separate issue.
4. *look to the future* – a board must have the longest vision of any part of the organisation and impart a forward-looking mentality to staff.
5. *look to the outside* – a board must realise that its organisation is apart from society but a part of society, and constantly form, nurture and reform strategic alliances with other organisations and groups. 'Standalone' organisations will go the way of the dodo.
6. *redefine its mandate* – Health Boards, for example, must increasingly act on the realisation that the ultimate owner, the Minister, wants

the public to have input and has devolved some aspects of ultimate ownership to consumers. Health Boards will, to an even greater extent, be required to be owners in trust for the Minister *and* the public.

7. *decide its floor, staff's ceiling* – governance is ownership in action. Owners can be as involved or uninvolved as they choose, within the constraints of relevant legislation. Boards must define (and redefine, as problems/situations/opportunities arise) their role in day-to-day activity, where they end and the Chief Executive Officer begins, how deep in the organisation they go, how high and close to ownership the Chief Executive Officer comes.

8. *separate the wheat from the chaff* – boards must separate issues that require the application of governance from those that do not.

9. *do the housekeeping* – a board agenda is the board's agenda. Members must agree when, how often and for how long they will meet, what they will discuss and what information they need.

10. *have pride* – good governance empowers organisations to produce good effects in society. Board members need to have pride in their work.

Ends-focused governance, means-focused operations

A major feature of this new governance is a better understanding of what 'policy-making' is and what it is not. Policy-making is authoritative empowerment. It is the act of continuously refining and adding to the written body of board values, values which determine the range of possible decisions a Chief Executive Officer has at her disposal for any given issue. The core policy of a board is its Mission Statement, the careful articulation of its desired effect on society, clarified with and approved by the owner(s) in whose trust the board acts. The board's Mission Statement is the launching pad for all action. Thus policy-making has its beginnings in desired effects and is ends-inspired, whereas operational decision-making is means-inspired and begins at the point where the board feels that its policy articulation is sufficiently specific to empower its Chief Executive Officer and staff.

By their nature, policies are, and look, different from operational documents. They must be brief, clear, living, forward-looking, centrally held and available to all. Operational documents are lengthy, detailed, shorter-term and activity-dominated. They do not require board approval because they are consistent with policy. Too often, boards mistake operational documents brought to them for approval for policy documents. In the absence of the kind of policy-making promoted here, these documents, if they contain any diamonds of policy, have buried them in a pile of the less precious stones of operations. They will not be recognised or remembered; they are brought to the board by staff and, once approved, removed by staff. Any board member, asked what constitutes the body of board policy, should be able to produce a slim file of documents that have had life breathed into them by the debate that is governance. Instead, given current board dysfunction, such a request would probably result in the member contacting the Chief Executive Officer and the latter supplying mounds of operational manuals and plans. Painful sifting would reveal dead, stillborn, new and old policies, many conflicting with each other.

I have said that policy looks different from operation. Examples may help. A small organisation, a family (board) decides that it wants to achieve a holiday annually. This constitutes a policy (ends). It decides that this policy is not yet explicit enough to empower the Travel Agent (Chief Executive Officer). Further debate results in progression of the family policy-making; it is decided that the holiday will be in winter, for two weeks, in a warm climate, by the sea, at a total cost of no more than £1,500. The board is now prepared to accept any reasonable implementation (means) by its Chief Executive Officer. If the board wishes to be more specific, it may ('we want Italy and we want self-catering'). The Chief Executive Officer does not have an office organised into divisions such as the Warm Division, the £1,500 Division, the Fortnight Division, etc. Indeed, her office may be organised along lines that are incomprehensible and of no interest to the Board, such as Finance, Personnel, Airlines, Affiliates, Legal, etc. Here is the crux: how could the family possibly end up with the holiday it wanted if presented with choices couched in such operational language and detail? As another example, how could a family cause a home to be built if the only decisions it was consulted about concerned wires, bricks, pipes and glass? Facile as these analogies may look, many boards function poorly, precisely because they approve means rather that decide ends. Health Boards suffer more than most, given the difficulty in articulation of ends, a difficulty exceeded only by the paramount importance of this articulation. Concentration on means orphans a board from the parenthood of mission and its derived ends-focused policies. At best, such a board sits atop an organisation brimful of activity that is intermittently and incompletely under its control and producing ends both desired and undesired. Boards that decide to engage in governance as promoted here will discover the power of policy-making and miss the old way of doing things as much as PC-users miss typewriters; the change will be that revolutionary.

The boundaries of governance and policy layering

Policy comes in layers, the topmost being the Mission Statement, lower layers being increasingly specific, each layer being completely contained by the layer above it. The top layer is the end of the external owner's involvement, the take-off point for governance. The bottom layer is the end of the board's involvement, the take-off point for the Chief Executive Officer. Consider the following progression of fictional policy.

- *The South-Western Health Authority will strive to promote and produce the maximum health status of the population it serves, through the efficient use of its resources* [a sentence from a Mission Statement perhaps six sentences in length].
- *Access to services will be equitable* [a sentence from a sub-policy, also brief, perhaps subsidiary to the 'efficient use of resources' phrase in the Mission Statement and articulated by the board to make it clear that efficiency should not be achieved at the expense of poor access to services because of geographic location, mobility, etc.].
- *Specific provisions will be made to ensure that care is delivered as close to the consumer's home as is feasible, and no less than 45% of total revenue will be allocated for this* [a sub-policy directing the Chief Executive Officer to lean as far as the board deems possible to community-based care].
- *50% of community funding will be specifically directed at services for the elderly* [greater specificity in policy].
- *Community-based services for the elderly will be weighted in favour of those living alone, by allocating 35% of the pertinent resources* [even greater specificity].

The excerpts above are from fictional policies. They are not great: how could they be, given that they are the product not of collective wisdom but only of what passes for mine? None the less, they show a relentless march from mission (ends) towards, but not as far as, operations (means). The layers of policy progress from 'maximum health status' to equitable access to community-based care to services for the elderly to services for the elderly who are living alone. The board will continually refine and clarify the policies; the total volume will never be big (50 pages?) but the Chief Executive Officer will always know within what range of decisions he is empowered, where his creativity can begin and at what sub-decision crossroads he can empower his staff. The organisation is focused on ends.

A further, shorter example of policy-layering:

- *The hospital will care for patients with dedicated and competent staff* [mission]
- *Recruitment practices will be non-discriminatory and staff's potential will be continually developed* [policy]
- *Staff development activity will foster a patient-focused interdisciplinary approach to care* [sub-policy]
- *Patient focus will be assured through active gauging of levels of satisfaction etc.* [sub-sub-policy].

Again, there is progressive clarification of policy, starting at the Mission Statement. The policies above 'contain' the policies below. The language does not constrain staff; it tells them where their creativity must begin. The board controls without meddling. Staff know exactly what work the board has done (policies are available to all), as opposed to being unclear as to whether the board did anything at all other than rubber stamp some weighty tomes of operational details.

Board policies can be organised in a handful of categories. One of these is ends, as discussed above. While there will be a lesser concentration on means, there needs to be some and there can be a category for this also. Policies in this category are also derived from the Mission Statement and express, with layered specificity, the values, ethics and principles the board requires of its Chief Executive Officer in dealing with staff. A board that approaches policy-making in this manner will spend a long time discussing, for example, the principles it wishes to guide its Chief Executive Officer in resolving staff grievances, and no time at all approving a lengthy 'personnel grievances resolution policy'. The latter will be merely the detailed reasonable interpretation by the Chief Executive Officer of the board's direction, policy layers in this area having been developed as far as the board felt appropriate.

Another policy category will be 'board–CEO relationship'. If the policies therein are perfect, the following will never happen.

1. The Chief Executive Officer makes a decision and the board takes her to task because it wanted to be the decision-maker on that issue.
2. The board makes a decision and the Chief Executive Officer protests that this issue was not a board matter.
3. The Chief Executive Officer asks the board for a decision on a matter it wanted to leave up to her.
4. The board asks the Chief Executive Officer to decide on a matter she feels to be a board function.

The policies will never be perfect, of course, but constantly tending them is a powerful activity and contrasts with the *ad hoc*ism so rampant in current governance, where board–CEO issues are resolved as they arise but rarely used to refine the relationship or add to a body of policy. The implications for management are enormous. Since policies are available to all, staff know what decisions managers are empowered to make and managers know the point, on any issue, at which the board has allowed the CEO to get creative. Staff activity will be characterised by clarity of purpose, knowledge of limits and the expectation of creativity.

A few other policy categories can be created, such as Board Process – how the board itself will do business. It is unlikely that a board will find use for more than half a dozen policy categories, and because of layering and the constant upkeep of policy, every board member can be familiar with every sentence of the brief but powerful body of board work.

Consider the current Waiting List Initiative. Admittedly, government conceived and decreed it, but Health Boards have embraced it and so it will be respectfully commented on here as an example of questionable governance in light of policy-making as described above.

A Waiting List Initiative buys surgical activity. Several critical governance issues should be resolved before such a specific operational decision is made. Is a Waiting List Initiative consistent with equity of access? Perhaps it discriminates against those with medical as opposed to surgical conditions. If the elderly or women or travellers are under-represented, it may discriminate against them. If Community Care staff have to provide post-discharge follow-up etc., a proportion of the Waiting List Initiative monies should be allocated to them, otherwise they will have to divert from others. What is the validity of a waiting list? Although it is quantitative, how accurate is it? Is there satisfaction that alternatives to surgery have been maximally used? If these critical governance issues have been dealt with and a Waiting List Initiative still appears desirable, there is no problem. If they have not, we are still at the stage of profoundly flawed governance.

One of the attractions of a Waiting List Initiative is that it is easy to measure its effects. It will always be easier to measure activity than evaluate results, to count means rather than evaluate ends. This should not seduce boards away from the articulation of policies that are ends-focused. Crude measurement of clear ends is better than precise measurements of mere means. Further, boards need to look carefully at every issue and ask the initial critical questions. Is this a policy matter? If it isn't, what is it doing here? Let us discuss with the Chief Executive Officer the lack of clarity in our policies that caused her to bring the issue here, and amend accordingly. If it is a policy matter, let us look at our existing policies to see where this issue fits and decide on it in a way that is consistent with them; we can alter policy a little if we deem it necessary. Let us then ask the Chief Executive Officer if she is clear as to the range within which she has freedom to operate in this matter. We can go home then.

Conclusion

Governance as espoused here requires board discipline and processes that constantly focus members on the wood as opposed to the trees. It will take time and will require a national focus on the nature of governance, with attendant debate, education and research. Formal orientation and continuing education of board members has to begin, and this challenge can be taken up by such bodies as the IPA. That it should happen can be adopted as process policy by boards themselves. We need to explode the myth that boards not composed of 'experts' cannot govern: they can, usually better, because a focus on ends is within the grasp of all reasonable people who accept their collective ownership role when sitting on boards.

We need to clarify the trusteeship given to boards. If the public are to be more involved in Health Boards, channels need to open to assure public input in framing the Mission Statement. Whether doctors are to be regarded as an internal consumer group or an advisory group, it will be necessary that medical staff have formal structures to ensure that the board hears that voice clearly and at first hand without abdicating its governance role. Some brave government will agree to review the composition of boards for appropriateness, but fundamental change need not and cannot wait for this. Good governance will beget better governance. As always, the first steps will be the most difficult but the journey will be worth it, particularly in healthcare.

PART THREE

Funding

CHAPTER 5

Healthcare – the Context

Miriam Hederman O'Brien

Introduction

What significant contribution can a layperson make to a book on managing healthcare in Ireland? As the readers will have more expert knowledge than the writer, the most useful approach is to state some of the questions which occur to an outsider who is a user of the product and has been an interested observer for many years of the Irish health services. These questions may appear naïve to the health professionals. The answers, however, could possibly help non-professionals to assess the quality of the health services and understand the direction in which policy is taking them. The questions, basic as they are, might even provide a certain context for the discussions of the experts.

Why spend money on healthcare?

It is almost universally accepted that money should be spent on national health budgets and that these budgets are likely to grow. However, other budgets, such as those providing for the environment, housing, employment, education and even the enforcement of justice, may have a wider impact and a better effect on the population's quality of health than the same money spent in traditional areas of healthcare. It is natural that we, as electors, should want government to provide the structures needed for civilised living, including healthcare services. As taxpayers, we want to focus spending on where it is most effective. We do not want to face up to an 'either or' situation in relation to vital services: housing versus a hospital, or waste disposal versus a prison. But we do understand (even though we may be reluctant to acknowledge) the idea that, in reality, resources are finite and choices must be made.

In the debate which normally precedes decisions on priorities, competing claims are considered but the relative impact of different kinds of spending is rarely examined. It is not easy to evaluate this impact; in order to reach the best conclusion, a combination of scientific analysis, social judgement, economic assessment and international experience is required. Since I do not have the necessary qualifications, I merely raise some questions about the national environment in which we frame our policy and hope that those who are more qualified will provide the appropriate solutions.

If a visitor from Mars were to prepare a report on the problems of Earth, he/she/it would identify many areas where the lack of money to spend on health services is depriving the people of the opportunity to lead dignified and useful lives and preventing their country from achieving economic progress. This is such a serious barrier that the International Monetary Fund now specifically includes it in its approach to countries of the Developing World. Children are afflicted by diseases which could easily be cured; adults are incapacitated by lack of treatment and are unable to provide for themselves and their families; young parents die before they can rear their families. These countries are spending too little on healthcare services because they do not have financial resources or because the few resources they have are being applied to the provision of arms or are dissipated in other ways.

At the other extreme, the countries of the 'North' (i.e. the highly developed and wealthy nations, among which Ireland must be included) use an increasing percentage of national wealth for the provision of healthcare. The governments in these states are concerned as to whether they can sustain such expenditure and whether they will have sufficient resources to meet the bills for other priorities. It does not matter particularly whether the finances come from private or public funds if spending on health becomes a cuckoo in the national nest, forcing out other birds such as education, employment, security, and investment in enterprise and social progress.

The increasing age of the population, with the consequent need for more money to provide for medical care for the elderly, when allied to the development of more expensive drugs and procedures, provides a picture of progressively increasing healthcare budgets. These, in turn, could lead to declining general standards of health *if the necessary basic social structures are not properly established and maintained.* In other words, we cannot ignore the extent to which our health is affected by our social and physical environment. This applies to every income group, but particularly to the poor.

One of the most challenging studies of income distribution and poverty in *developed* countries is that of Richard Wilkinson in *Unhealthy Societies*. In Wilkinson's opinion, once societies reach a certain level of economic development – around an average annual income of $3,000 per head – health and mortality tend to be increasingly influenced by changes in the relative position of groups within the society. The extent to which a community is 'comfortable' with itself appears to affect the physical and mental well-being of its component parts. Social solidarity and reasonably equal income distribution are not the same thing, but they are clearly related. If Wilkinson's arguments are valid (and they are certainly persuasive), neither the total amount spent on health services nor the availability of sophisticated procedures will, of itself, offset the decreasing health standards and mortality rates of those at the bottom of widening income differentials in a prosperous society.

It is unnecessary to remind the readers of this book that one of the major problems in assessing standards of health is the extent to which the providers define the product and the recipients express their satisfaction (or otherwise) in this area. It is therefore always difficult to justify our spending as being the most effective. If we were to reward family doctors for the number of healthy people on their lists, we would provide a significant incentive to save money, possibly at the expense of adequate medical care; furthermore, the health statistics might look better than the reality. The other extreme is an approach to healthcare which would utilise every available procedure until the budget runs out and then declare a state of emergency and be unable to provide quite basic services until a new financial year.

The reasons for spending taxpayers' money (and our own private funds) on healthcare are complex. They include altruism (we have a duty to all our citizens and a greater duty to those who are in greater need), pragmatism (if people are not healthy they cannot work; they will be poor and unable to contribute to the economy) and self-interest (each one of us feels pain and fears the onset of illness and death; a 'pool' of disease in the community cannot be contained and may affect us). These considerations contribute to create a base of social solidarity for the strategic organisation of health services.

How should we spend on healthcare?

How do we expect policy-makers to find the correct balance of expenditure on the various aspects of healthcare? The recent *Management Development Strategy in the Health and Personal Social Services in Ireland* Report to the Minister for Health (November 1996) contains comprehensive recommendations to:

- improve the recruitment, selection and initial training of health personnel
- introduce performance measurement across health authorities and ally it to the allocation of resources
- develop the careers of health professionals
- increase management education in the health services.

An office has already been established to implement the recommendations. The issue of 'managing' the health services is therefore now high on the policy agenda.

Three elements contribute to a good equilibrium in the use of resources. The first is a combination of *expert opinion* and independent judgement within the decision-making process itself. The healthcare experts are required for their special knowledge and because they will be responsible for delivering the policy. Competent people, not professionally involved in delivering healthcare, are needed to evaluate the arguments from a background of non-medical expert knowledge and to ensure that the needs of other areas and other interests are taken into account.

The second element is the *training* of healthcare personnel. The quality of care depends to such a large extent on the quality of the people who give it – not only on their dedication and competence but also on their approach to making the service as effective as possible – that it is impossible to overestimate the importance of their training. Such training has long been acknowledged as being necessary on a continuing basis, but other pressures intervene and it has had to take its place in the queue of competing demands. The strategy now being adopted should bring about a significant improvement in this area. The education of healthcare professionals must also provide an understanding of the wider aspects of their work: the 'social solidarity' to which they should contribute.

The third element which contributes to the best use of resources is *relevant, focused research*. Such research is of two kinds: first, the study of the best way of delivering services (which will be a responsibility of the Health Services Management Centre); second, the identification of areas of need for primary or applied research in an Irish context (to which we will return later).

If we accept the three elements outlined above as contributing to the most effective use of resources, we can apply them to the situation in Ireland.

Expert opinion – the combination of medical and non-medical experts

The forging of a team spirit between medical and non-medical experts has been a difficult accomplishment in every country, in every age. It has worked best when there has been a sense of common urgency and common interest. It is therefore necessary to persuade the suppliers of healthcare of the urgency of the need to manage the spending of health budgets in Ireland more effectively. The approach of the state, as the main funder, is very important but the health providers must be convinced of the advantages of becoming more involved in that management process. The role of the health insurers in this area is currently under-utilised and has been confused in the public mind by the travails of the VHI. The controversy that arose about the status of BUPA has also diverted attention away from the positive contribution which health insurers can make to the quality of the health service, if they approach the issue in the interests of their clients/subscribers.

The *Report of the Commission on Health Funding*, published in 1989, made many recommendations which have been implemented, and the official response to this and more recent reports can be found in *Shaping a Healthier Future - A strategy for effective healthcare in the 1990s*, issued by the Department of Health in 1994.

Having identified some of the problems which existed at that time, including 'confusions of political and executive functions', 'imbalance between national and local decision-making', 'absence of a role for evaluation', 'inadequate accountability', 'insufficient integration of related services' and 'inadequate representation of service users', the Commission on Health Funding proposed a new administrative structure. Alternatives to the existing structure are examined at some length in Chapter 9 of the Report, and the reasons for preferring the proposed Health Services Executive Authority are outlined. It would be the task of such an Authority to harness the combined energies of the medical and non-medical experts in order to achieve the best possible health service. The Health (Amendment) Act 1996, the current restructuring of health services in Dublin, Kildare and Wicklow, and the Management Development Strategy already referred to should help to address many of the problems identified in the Commission' s Report, albeit in a different way.

As the Commission considered the various sectors of the healthcare services it became increasingly evident that the *providers* of the services – general practitioners, community and hospital nurses, consultants and hospital doctors, health educators, pharmacists, dentists, physiotherapists and other specialists – should share the responsibility for the management of resources with the professional managers of the health services. Such involvement would be welcomed by some providers and painful for others. However, encouragement of clinical personnel to become more expert in the management aspects of their work has been shown to yield good results in terms of patient care. It has been adopted as an approach in *Shaping a Healthier Future*, which rests on three principles: equity, quality of service and accountability.

> Regardless of the level of resources which can be made available, we need to look more closely at how we use them. It will be clear throughout the Health Strategy that a central element in the planned reshaping of the services is the emphasis which will in future be placed on achieving the greatest benefit from whatever resources are available. (*Shaping a Healthier Future*, p. 12)

This document states that 'The Department of Health will no longer be involved in the detailed management of the health services'. Such a decision requires the *acceptance of responsibility* by those who organise and deliver the services, and greater emphasis on the *policy* role of the Department.

The experience of the UK in restructuring the delivery of health services has been divisive, but it has given us in Ireland examples of what we might adopt and what we should exclude. With regard to the general medical scheme (GMS) contract, which was negotiated as the Commission on Health Funding prepared its Report, I quote from Chapter 11.

We note that the new contract is more flexible than its predecessor since it is subject to periodic review, and any changes agreed upon can be readily implemented. *The present agreement should therefore be regarded as an interim arrangement to which changes may be made in the light of experience rather than as an unalterable final version.* (11.43, p. 218; emphasis added)

The interaction between hospital and non-hospital healthcare services has far-reaching implications not only for the funding of both sectors but also for the recipients of the services. Given the current clinical workload of many nurses and doctors, it is easy to understand why they have little time or enthusiasm for 'management' meetings. Yet, without a significant improvement in the management of resources – including their own time – they will have to suffer arbitrary changes. It has been recognised that the present situation, even with the partial progress that has been made, cannot continue indefinitely.

Training

Basic medical professional education: There is a general view in this country that the quality of our healthcare providers is among the best in the world. It would be a brave commentator who would suggest that we have our share of average, and even below-average performers, but the disparity of medical treatment which is revealed from time to time is an indication that the quality of the providers of that treatment is not equal. In a different context, the arguments of the nursing profession in favour of early retirement are another indication that a problem exists. The serious debate which is taking place on the curriculum of students of every branch of medicine is a sign that those in charge of medical education are aware of the problems they face.

With knowledge expanding in all areas of medical science, how widely can students be trained without overloading them to such an extent that they receive only a superficial or even transitory knowledge of basic principles? Which subjects should be studied after graduation and which should remain in the core curriculum?

This is not a subject that can be dealt with adequately in this chapter, but the structural issue of the number of training centres for medical personnel in Ireland, and the effects that this has on their separate resources (including the range of experts available at any single centre), must be raised. If our visitor from Mars were to examine the population and size of Ireland, including Northern Ireland, in the context of the health needs of the people, how many schools of medical education and how much rationalisation in providing facilities for specialities would he/she/it recommend? Some implicit questions underlie the expensive training of highly skilled people. Are all those capable of pursuing such training, and anxious to pursue it, entitled to do so? If access is limited, as is the case in most countries, is it also confined to numbers required by the economy providing the cost of the training? The Irish system appears to have answered 'no' to both questions, but the issue of the number accepted remains open. Needs are changing, both in Ireland and in the rest of the world, and the provision of medical training must reflect those needs.

Internship for newly qualified doctors, as currently operated, must be a subject for review. Without undertaking a profound analysis of this issue, an outsider would wonder why the newly qualified doctors are not allocated places on a basis which reflects their needs and abilities and the national requirements of the medical services. The strangely steep pyramid which is found in the staff structure of some departments, particularly outside the city hospitals, means that a consultant may arrive in his/her department to find a completely fresh team of newly qualified doctors in attendance once or even twice a year.

Further and specialised medical professional education: This area is probably less sensitive than might be expected because of the tradition of movement to other countries and centres for postgraduate research and training. There is also an understanding of the need for periodic 'updating' which has spread from other professions and will be extended among the providers of healthcare services. *Further* training involves refresher courses of varying duration, but it may also include improving skills which were not specifically part of the basic training of the professionals involved. Management involvement, mentioned above, will be easier for those who obtain a grasp of the vocabulary and fundamentals of professional management. Communication skills, which most professionals, particularly at senior level, believe they possess, have been shown to be less than satisfactory in many areas of the healthcare services. These skills must be improved in the interests of patients, the public and the professionals concerned. Evaluation of treatments and products which have become routine is necessary in every profession. How much is spent by pharmaceutical manufacturers, for example, in developing and promoting their products and how much in providing independent assessment of their relative efficacy? Given the cost of research, it is understandable that the drug companies spend very much more than the regulators. But is the balance correct? Where such independent assessments have been made, they must then be brought to the attention of the users.

There are many other areas in which 'further training' is necessary and available. One of the principal effects of a good, multidisciplinary programme of such training is the knowledge it brings to each speciality of the changes taking place in others. Because of the pressures of their daily work, some clinicians do not appear to be fully aware of the current educational programme of the nurses who take care of their patients. Pharmacologists and busy family doctors, both already in the front-line of patient contact, could assist each other to a far greater extent if they shared occasional joint information sessions. The list of potential benefits can be extended into every aspect of healthcare.

Specialised further education has traditionally involved movement from one centre to another. Promotion normally requires special qualifications; the increasing specialisation of medicine itself accelerates the trend. However, specialisation also impinges on the delivery of services. An exasperated Chief Executive Officer of a Health Board recently complained that, with the current rate of specialisation, he would soon have to appoint consultants for left and right nostrils while he remained without a service for nose ailments. He exaggerated, of course, but his dilemma is not confined to his region or to Ireland; other countries have begun to try to find solutions which ensure wider expertise without imperilling the improvements which specialisation has brought to the practice of medicine.

To illustrate some current needs for specialisation, I refer to an important section of the *Report of the Expert Group on the Blood Transfusion Service Board* (1995) which has received little public comment. The Group recommended that:

> the Blood Transfusion Service Board should develop more fully into a Centre for Transfusion Medicine which would have clearly defined medical, teaching and research functions as well as its current role in operating a blood transfusion service. This would not diminish the importance of its existing functions, rather it would emphasise the side dimensions involved in the expanding field of transfusion medicine. (4.49, p. 73)

The Report goes on to suggest steps which should be taken to strengthen the BTSB's capacity to 'play a leading role in the promotion of research and development in transfusion medicine in Ireland'. Those steps include an improved structure, more scientific staff, particularly at doctoral level, increasing the complement of consultant staff available, and the development of much closer 'day to day links with the haematology departments of Irish hospitals' (4.64, p. 76).

The Report welcomed an initiative by the Cork Blood Transfusion Centre with the Regional and Mercy Hospitals in Cork for a training post at registrar level, and encouraged the increase of links with medical schools. Whatever forms these links may take with hospitals and medical schools, the Group stated that:

> it is crucial that BTSB medical personnel remain up to date with developments in their field, both locally and internationally, and that they act as a conduit for information to their hospital colleagues. (4.66, p. 76)

The issue of making choices was raised above, and it is clear that developments in one area of medicine will require contraction in others. More resources in transfusion medicine will have to be justified by more efficacious treatment, better prevention, and improved medical results in related areas. I have quoted from this Report because it illustrates the policy changes towards greater integration of research, development and treatment which should take place. Having been involved in its preparation, I regret that, despite the continued and wide coverage of some of its findings, this important area has been largely ignored.

Research

The State facilitates investment in research through its support of universities and research institutions (including hospitals) and the favourable tax treatment of private investment in research. The argument about the level and extent of such investment must be pursued elsewhere.

It has been contended that a small country without large, well-endowed centres of scientific excellence cannot compete in primary research. Irish research institutions should therefore co-operate as partners in larger projects on basic research, when they can identify a specific aspect in which they are competent. It can also be argued that they should put much of their resources into evaluating international research and applying it to national conditions. But we need to ensure that primary research takes place, if only to safeguard the quality of our teaching and training. There is certainly room to increase existing Irish research co-operation within the European framework in both basic and applied research.

In the Nordic countries, there is a greater degree of co-ordination in health, as in other services, than is found elsewhere in Europe. Patients can be sent to a centre of expertise in any Nordic country, and experts of one nationality may specialise in another country: this is partially mirrored, informally, within these islands. It is not, however, taken into account when Irish – or British – policy-makers are deciding how to allocate resources. It is not even officially considered within the boundaries of the island of Ireland, other than for dealing with a catastrophe, as far as I know.

On the purely national plane it is worthy of comment that there has been little official direct state investment in research in areas which have been identified as being in the interest of the national health. If, for example, we could delay the onset of immobility and mental confusion in the elderly by even an average of five years, we would improve the quality of life of the old to a significant extent and we would also reduce the cost of their medical care. It might be expected, therefore, that the state itself would fund research into these and similar areas which would affect the healthcare of a considerable section of the population. This has been done in the recently launched National Cancer Strategy, where a clinical research unit (within the Health Research Board) will focus on clinical research to:

- provide an infrastructure for a multidisciplinary, multi-institutional approach to clinical cancer research
- focus on clinical research in a way that contributes to the knowledge and treatment of the most common cancers in Ireland
- assist participation in collaborative research with other countries, and in particular EU countries and co-operative groups.

This strategy might be fruitfully extended to other areas.

The appropriate method of delivering healthcare has been identified as contributing to the effectiveness and efficiency of the service. The Department of Health has commissioned work in this area and has itself undertaken assessments. The *Report of the Commission on Health Funding* dwelt at considerable length on the need for continuing research in this area, and advocated that 'a multi-disciplinary Department of Health Services Research should be established within an Irish university' (10.54, p. 194).

Clinical research can have implications for healthcare costs and treatments: developments in treating chronic or formerly fatal illnesses, for example, could have a considerable impact on long-term care needs. New drugs can enable patients to recuperate at home or away from acute hospitals, with consequential effects on the distribution of resources.

To quote again from the *Report of the Commission on Health Funding*, in the section on the proposed Health Services Executive Authority, dealing with its role in research:

> In all areas of research, the Authority would be guided by priorities given to it by the Minister for Health. This would ensure that the limited resources which are available for health research would be channelled into areas most likely to produce the greatest benefits for the health services as a whole. (10.50, p. 194)

The role of the Health Research Board, which currently promotes, commissions and conducts medical, health and health services research on a national level, would be enhanced, although its structure might be changed, in the context of an active policy of state-funded research as outlined above.

Epidemiological research is closely related to the information and evaluation which is needed for the day-to-day management of the health services. Clinical research is necessary for academic institutions, teaching and hospitals. Health services research should affect the policy agenda, monitor international findings and evaluate the current usage and level of health services in Ireland.

The future

No objective rules exist to determine the appropriate amount of spending on health services. International comparisons merely show that richer countries spend more, both absolutely and relatively, than poorer countries. The standard of healthcare reflects the values and culture of a community, the quality of its healthcare personnel, and environmental and other factors.

Planning for the future healthcare needs of the Irish people depends on forecasts of the demographic structure, likely clinical developments, environmental threats, changes in behaviour and contingency plans for 'unforeseen' calamities. In other words, it is an essential, high-skill, high-risk enterprise.

We should be concerned not only about the health of individuals, including of course ourselves, but also about the general health of the population around us. The 'environment' for health purposes includes not only the structure of the health services available but the physical conditions in which we live, the impact of new threats to health throughout the world, and the promise of new remedies and new treatments for old diseases and intractable illness. People are being made aware that they can affect their own health and that of those around them by their patterns of behaviour. Expectations are high and growing.

The most constructive approach to good healthcare services is a combination of access to effective delivery at the local level and co-operation in the high-technological, highly scientific procedures at national and international level.

I hope that the experts will hatch out a health service which will be a cause for praise rather than being either a starveling or a voracious cuckoo in the national nest.

CHAPTER 6

Health Funding and Expenditure in Ireland

Fergal Lynch

Introduction

The most appropriate level of public and private funds to be allocated to healthcare has been the subject of international debate for decades. Health spending as a proportion of national income has risen enormously in virtually every developed country since the 1960s, but it remains very difficult to judge whether the increased resources have yielded proportionate improvements in healthcare or in the health of individuals. This chapter examines the main trends in Irish health expenditure since the 1960s. It considers alternative sources of funding for healthcare, including the question of greater private funding or revised approaches to public funding. Next, the chapter examines the process by which decisions are made regarding allocation of resources between different healthcare providers (such as health boards, hospitals and voluntary agencies), and notes in particular the attempt to move away from incremental approaches to resource allocation. Finally, some future issues connected with health funding and expenditure are considered – it is suggested that the most immediate challenge will be to evaluate the outcomes as opposed to the outputs of spending on healthcare.

Trends in Irish health spending

In common with most other developed countries, Ireland has experienced a substantial increase in health expenditure since the early 1960s. However, there was a significant break in this trend for a period in the late 1980s due to a programme of sustained reduction in public spending. It is convenient to examine the trends in health spending by reference to (a) spending from public health sources and (b) spending from private sources. Total spending on health services in Ireland is then considered.

Public health spending in Ireland

Table 6.1 provides details of spending from public sources on the Irish health services for selected years since 1960. The *current prices* show the actual (or nominal) amount of money that was spent in that year. Obviously, these have little meaning in comparative terms unless price changes over the period are taken into account. The current prices are therefore shown in *constant terms at 1990 prices*. One method of taking account of price differences would be to use inflation figures (such as the Consumer Price Index) to show how health expenditure had risen or fallen in real terms. However, ordinary inflation data such as those generated by the Consumer Price Index are not a particularly good indicator of medical inflation. There is no official health services price index in Ireland, but there is an implicit deflator contained in the National Accounts (Public Authorities' Net Current Expenditure series) which can be applied as a reasonable indicator of real trends in health expenditure.

Using this deflator, and taking 1960 as the reference year, it can be seen from Table 6.1 that Irish public health spending almost doubled between 1960 and 1970, trebled up to 1975 and more than quadrupled between 1960 and 1980. It then held constant until 1988, when it fell noticeably in real terms. It did not recover to its earlier position until 1991. By 1995, the latest year for which all of the data required for calculating the index are available, public health spending had exceeded five times its 1960 level using this measure.

Private health spending

In addition to the public spending on healthcare described above, there is substantial expenditure from private sources each year. However, details of some elements of private health expenditure are difficult to obtain and it is necessary to make estimates based on the information available. Table 6.2 gives details of estimated private health spending for selected years up to 1995.

Expenditure on private health insurance (VHI was the only insurer available to the general public during the period under review) is the only item which can be quoted with certainty; the other elements are based on estimates of private spending from the CSO National

Table 6.1. Trends in public health spending (selected years, 1960–1996)

Year	1960	1970	1975	1980	1987	1988	1989
Current prices (£m)	19.5	72.8	242.6	701.0	1,221.5	1,231.5	1,318.0
Constant (1990) prices (£m)	353.4	673.2	1,076.9	1,490.7	1,404.5	1,359.4	1,384.9
Index (1960 = 1)	1.0	1.9	3.0	4.2	4.0	3.8	3.9

Year	1990	1991	1992	1993	1994	1995	1996
Current prices (£m)	1,463.9	1,631.0	1,829.7	2,016.6	2,145.8	2,298.9	2,354.2
Constant (1990) prices (£m)	1,463.9	1,523.9	1,629.1	1,692.6	1,751.1	1,833.7	n/a
Index (1960 = 1)	4.1	4.3	4.6	4.8	5.0	5.2	n/a

Source: Revised Estimates for Public Services. Index derived from CSO data.

Table 6.2. Estimated private health expenditure (£m), selected years 1984–1995

	1984	1987	1990	1993	1994	1995
VHI expenditure	92.6	150.1	171.1	203.1	223.6	247.7
Household expenditure	201.4	231.1	277.0	347.6	357.6	371.7
Non-household expenditure	4.6	5.0	6.1	8.0	8.5	9.1
Capital expenditure	12.9	37.5	42.0	32.7	39.9	55.0
Total	311.5	423.7	496.2	591.4	629.6	683.5

Note: Estimates of non-household expenditure are extrapolated from estimates by Tussing (1985) in respect of 1980 in line with trends in current Department of Health expenditure.
Source: Department of Health and CSO data.

Accounts. These are drawn from the Household Budget Survey and supplemented by data from a variety of other sources.

The largest element of the CSO estimates is in respect of expenditure by households on such items as the fees of doctors, dentists and opticians, hospital charges, and drugs and medicines. Refunds from the public system in respect of any of these charges are excluded from Table 6.2 to avoid double counting. The CSO also supplies estimates of private capital spending on healthcare, including expenditure on equipping private hospitals and surgeries. Finally, Table 6.2 includes tentative estimates of other private non-household expenditure. This relates to a small number of employment-based health insurance schemes for which very few expenditure data are available.

Estimates of overall health expenditure

Subject to the qualifications above regarding estimates of private health expenditure, data on estimated overall health spending from both public and private sources are presented in Table 6.3. For completeness, these estimates include certain elements that do not appear in the Department of Health's allocation, but which are clearly related to health services. These include European Social Fund expenditure on training programmes for the disabled, expenditure from the National Lottery on health projects, and Treatment Benefits for dental, optical and aural services operated by the Department of Social Welfare.

In Table 6.3, public and private expenditure are expressed as a proportion of Gross Domestic Product (GDP) and Gross National Product (GNP). It is usual to express health expenditure as a share of GDP. However, in Ireland there is now a large divergence between GDP and GNP, due largely to interest payments on foreign borrowings which are deducted (along with other payments) to calculate GNP. This suggests that GNP would be a better indicator of the extent to which health services absorb the resources actually available to the Irish economy.

It can be seen that when measured in terms of national income, total Irish health expenditure has fluctuated between 7.5% and 9% of GDP and between 8.4% and 10.2% of GNP during the past 15 years. Within these figures, private health spending has tended to remain at between 1.7% and 2.0% of national income, while public health spending has shown a somewhat wider variation.

The trends indicated by this measure illustrate that expressing health expenditure as a proportion of national income is perhaps not a very satisfactory indicator of the level of funding available to the health services: the recent strength of economic growth in Ireland (i.e. increase in national income) means that health expenditure is being expressed as a proportion of an increasingly large figure. Thus even a significant real increase in health spending is not immediately

Table 6.3. Estimated overall health expenditure in Ireland (£m), selected years 1982–1995

	1982	1985	1988	1990	1991	1992	1993	1994	1995
Public (£m)	1,023	1,260	1,316	1,546	1,715	1,918	2,131	2,218	2,370
Private (£m)	230	353	459	496	532	576	591	630	684
Total (£m)	1,253	1,613	1,775	2,045	2,247	2,494	2,772	2,848	3,054
as % of GDP									
Public		7.6	7.1	5.9	5.7	6.1	6.4	6.5	6.4	6.1
Private		1.7	2.0	2.0	1.8	1.8	1.9	1.9	1.8	1.8
Total		9.3	9.1	7.9	7.5	7.9	8.3	8.4	8.2	7.9
as % of GNP									
Public		8.3	8.0	6.7	6.4	6.7	7.2	7.3	7.1	7.0
Private		1.7	2.2	2.3	2.0	2.1	2.1	2.2	2.0	2.0
Total		10.0	10.2	9.0	8.4	8.8	9.3	9.5	9.1	9.0

Source: Department of Health and CSO data.

Table 6.4. Estimated health spending in selected countries as a proportion of GDP, 1992–1995

Country	1992	1993	1994	1995
USA	14.0	14.3	14.3	14.5
Canada	10.3	10.2	9.8	9.5
Australia	8.7	8.6	8.5	8.4
France	9.4	9.8	9.7	9.9
Austria	8.9	9.4	9.7	9.6
Germany	9.3	9.3	9.5	9.6
Netherlands	8.8	9.0	8.8	8.8
Finland	9.3	8.8	8.3	8.2
Italy	8.5	8.6	8.3	7.7
Belgium	8.1	8.3	8.2	8.0
Ireland	**7.3**	**7.4**	**7.9**	**7.9**
Portugal	7.2	7.4	7.6	n/a
Spain	7.2	7.3	7.3	7.6
UK	7.0	6.9	6.9	6.9
Denmark	6.7	6.8	6.6	6.5
Luxembourg	6.3	6.2	5.8	n/a
Greece	4.5	4.6	5.2	n/a
Turkey	2.9	2.6	4.2	n/a

Source: Healthcare Reform: The Will to Change, Health Policy Studies, No. 8, OECD, Paris, 1996.

obvious when GNP rises at a higher rate. This is well illustrated by Tables 6.1 and 6.3. In Table 6.1 Irish health spending rose in real terms between 1993 and 1995 (from an index figure of 4.8 to 5.2), while in Table 6.3 it fell in terms of both GDP and GNP.

International health expenditure

Table 6.4 contains estimates by the Organisation for Economic Co-operation and Development (OECD) on overall health expenditure for EU member states and selected other countries. The data are not directly comparable to the Irish information in the tables above because, for purposes of valid comparison, the OECD uses a common definition of what constitutes health expenditure. This is necessary because not all countries classify their expenditure on a number of areas (e.g. child-care services, care of the elderly, training for the disabled) in the same way. Subject to this consideration and to the qualification above regarding the use of national income measures, it can be seen that Ireland's total health expenditure is broadly in line with that of most of its EU counterparts.

Sources of funding for healthcare

The growth in demand for health services (including a wide range of personal social services) has inevitably led to increasing pressure on the resources available. Apart from calls for extra funds from existing sources to be allocated to healthcare, questions have also been raised about the scope for new or alternative sources of funding for the health services. These questions generally centre around (a) 'untapped' or alternative methods and (b) increased private sources of funding. In relation to public funding, it is sometimes argued that a system of earmarked taxation, in which money is allocated to a dedicated fund for healthcare, would be a more satisfactory method of paying for health services. The 'social insurance' systems in some countries operate on this basis: there is a specified tax for healthcare from which all or part of the health services is funded. On the private side, it is argued that a compulsory system of health insurance for upper-income groups, while removing their entitlement to most or all publicly funded health services, would free up public money currently spent on those who could afford to pay for their own healthcare. It is argued that this money could then be reallocated to lower-income groups, thereby targeting resources at those most in need. Variations of this approach to greater private funding are advanced, but most centre on the question of either encouraging or compelling a designated upper-income category to take increasing responsibility for their health costs.

Public sources of funding

In Ireland over four-fifths of public funds for health services is voted directly from the Exchequer and comes from general taxation. A further 9% or so comes from health contributions, often known as the 'health levy', charged at 1.25% of income. The balance arises from public hospital charges for accommodation and other income, with a small element of receipts in respect of health services provided to residents of other EU member states. Table 6.5 gives details of these sources for 1996.

Table 6.5. Sources of funding for gross non-capital expenditure, 1996

Exchequer grants	83.0%
Health contributions	8.6%
Hospital charges and other income	6.1%
EU-related receipts	2.3%

Source: Department of Health.

When the Exchequer grants and health contributions are combined, it can be seen that over 90% of public funding for the health services in Ireland comes from general taxation. An alternative source of funding sometimes advocated for Ireland is a system based on the principles of social insurance such as those used in France and Germany. A social insurance system involves a direct payment to a fund designated for a specific purpose such as healthcare. Contributions to the fund can take account of ability to pay, and the lower income groups may have a contribution paid on their behalf by the state. Entitlement to publicly funded health services can then be dependent on contributions to the social insurance fund: those failing to contribute lose their eligibility for healthcare and may be charged for services accordingly.

The main arguments advanced in favour of such an 'earmarked' system of tax-funded healthcare in Ireland are that

- it would encourage consumers to make a close link between demands for health services and the cost of providing them
- it would safeguard the level of public funds available for health-care, particularly where there is pressure to reduce public spending as a whole
- it would help improve equity and efficiency, since both eligibility for services and the amount available for health spending would be determined by payments to the fund.

The Commission on Health Funding (1989) considered the case for and against an earmarked system of funding in some detail. It did not reach a unanimous conclusion, but the majority view was that the arguments for a separate health fund were not persuasive. Its report indicated that there was little empirical evidence either to support or to refute the argument that a separate health fund would lead to greater awareness of costs and a more responsible use of services by the general public. It concluded that

> it is difficult to assess whether awareness of the costs involved would, in practice, encourage people to be more economical in their use of the health services, since it is a common phenomenon of insurance that, having paid their premium, consumers tend to maximise their use of the cover provided (p. 88).

A majority of the Commission also argued against the case for insulating health services from competing pressures on public funds, pointing out that a similar case could be made on behalf of other areas of social expenditure such as education or income maintenance.

A further argument against the option of a dedicated health fund is that if it failed to cover the cost of health services for a full year it would have to be 'topped up' from another source, such as general taxation. It seems unlikely that a serious shortfall would be acceptable, and the pressure to make good the difference would be very strong.

Most decisions about allocation of resources to healthcare centre on marginal adjustments to the previous year's total. In other words, the debate focuses on the last few percentage points of the total money available for healthcare. If the health fund has to be topped up each year from another source, the real decision about the final total available for healthcare will be taken in the same way as in a general taxation system. Thus, the health fund fails in its attempts to 'insulate' the health services from other pressures on public spending.

The Commission on Health Funding felt that, if a separate health fund were to be established, it would have to be collected as part of the general income tax system since there would be significant administrative costs in setting up a separate means of collection. However, the Commission noted that 'this might reinforce the perception of the earmarked tax as being merely a part of income tax' (p. 89). Indeed, it pointed out that the existing health contribution was already essentially part of income tax since it was not allocated to a separate fund and did not determine eligibility for health services. The Commission recommended its abolition.

In summary, therefore, the most recent major independent review of sources of public funding for the health services in Ireland concluded, by majority opinion, that there was little to be gained from establishing a separate health fund. However, the fact that four members of the Commission on Health favoured such an approach suggests that it may attract further attention in the future.

Private sources of funding

As noted above, publicly funded health systems have been under continuing pressure to provide increasing levels and types of health service. Advances in treatment and care services have been more than matched by demands for ever more services from the public system. As publicly funded healthcare becomes subject to increasing expectations and rising costs, attention turns to alternative means of funding the demand through private sources.

One argument is that the public funds available for healthcare should be channelled towards the lower-income groups and that the highest income group should be required to make its own arrangements (most likely through private health insurance) to meet all or most of its healthcare costs. It is argued that this would have a positive redistributive impact, ensuring that public funds were directed towards those least able to make provision for their own healthcare.

Arguments for greater private funding of healthcare are usually linked to questions of eligibility for services: it is generally envisaged that an upper-income group would no longer be eligible for publicly funded services, making private arrangements effectively a necessity.

A variation of this approach is to retain eligibility for public services but to offer incentives to use privately funded healthcare. (It is important to emphasise that the focus here is on *funding* rather than *provision*: an upper-income group could continue using publicly provided health services, such as those in public hospitals, but they would be encouraged or compelled to pay from private sources, such as health insurance.)

The Commission on Health Funding examined the scope for a significantly greater private funding component in the Irish health services. Importantly, it noted that the choice at issue was that of a main funding model: a predominantly private system of health funding could be supplemented by some public funding, or vice versa. A majority of the Commission concluded that a predominantly private funding system for healthcare, under which a proportion of the population would be required to rely on their own resources, was not satisfactory. The majority expressed concern about equity, comprehensiveness of coverage and cost-effectiveness. In practical terms, those no longer entitled to publicly funded healthcare have to take out private health insurance. The majority of the Commission expressed concern that some of the more vulnerable groups, such as the elderly or chronically ill, would find it more costly to insure themselves. This argument remains valid today unless a community-rated system of health insurance (under which premiums are not calculated by reference to health risk factors) can be fully maintained. Otherwise those most in need of healthcare, even if in the upper-income category, would find it the most difficult to cover their own healthcare costs.

In addition to concerns about equity in a private funding model, concerns can be raised about comprehensiveness. The Commission on Health Funding was particularly conscious of practical difficulties in this regard. If private health insurance were made compulsory for a designated upper-income group (having removed or greatly reduced their public entitlement), the requirement would be difficult to enforce. Those failing to insure could hardly be refused vital treatment, or charged a full economic cost that they could not afford. On the other hand, a purely optional system of health insurance for those no longer entitled to publicly funded services would perhaps carry a safety-net that some might find difficult to ignore. 'The knowledge that treatment is unlikely to be refused makes purely optional health insurance impracticable' (Commission on Health Funding, p. 9).

Finally, the evidence available regarding the ability of privately based funding systems to control health costs did not inspire confidence among a majority of the Commission on Health Funding. Costs and per capita expenditure in the USA have risen at least as fast as those in predominantly public-funded health systems, and there appears to be little evidence of a noticeable improvement in this regard since the Commission reported. There have been some innovations among US insurers, including the development of close links between funders and providers (as in the case of Health Maintenance Organisations and various forms of 'preferred providers'). However, these initiatives have usually involved targeting low-risk, low-cost groups; the effect generally has been to *shift* rather than to *reduce* total costs. This is underlined by the fact that in 1995, US spending on healthcare as a proportion of GDP remained substantially higher than in most European countries which had predominantly publicly funded health systems (14.5% compared with a European average of 8.2%; OECD, 1996) and showed few signs of success in cost control from earlier years.

Since the Commission on Health Funding reported, concerns about equity, comprehensiveness of coverage and ability to control costs in a privately funded model (even for a specified upper income group) do not appear to have been alleviated. While calls for greater private responsibility for healthcare funding may be expected to continue, to date no comprehensive case has been presented showing how pressure on the public health system could be substantially reduced by an equitable, cost-effective private-based alternative.

Conclusion

The key conclusion to be drawn from the discussion above is that in Ireland no-one appears to have identified a source, whether public or private, that would offer significant additions to the resources available for healthcare. Privately based funding models do not appear to have addressed important shortcomings in equity, comprehensiveness and cost control, while changes to the tax system for public sources of funding such as a separate health fund would seem to make little difference to the amount collected or to public perceptions about its acceptability. In short, there is no 'crock of gold' for the Irish health services that has remained untapped. None the less, the debate about how best to fund health services will no doubt continue at home as well as internationally.

Resource allocation in healthcare

The previous section discussed the various potential sources of funding for healthcare. The next major question to be addressed is how these resources, however raised, are then to be allocated to the large range of competing providers such as hospitals, homes, community-based facilities and a range of social services. Irrespective of the amount raised and of the funding system(s) used, there will always be strong competition between healthcare providers for the available funds.

In the case of privately funded healthcare, the issue is perhaps a little less complex, because patients either pay out-of-pocket the 'market rate' charged by private providers (such as private hospitals or consultants in private practice) or draw upon private health insurance. In many cases private insurance companies (VHI and BUPA) have concluded agreements with hospitals and consultants on payments for private health services.

Resource allocation within the publicly funded healthcare system is somewhat more difficult, because the available funds must be divided between so many providers. For example, in 1996 there were 63 acute publicly funded hospitals (including maternity and paediatric hospitals), 42 long-stay district hospitals, 53 homes and 342 community residences for the mentally handicapped and a range of other bodies under the aegis of the Minister for Health (including advisory, professional and service providers). Some of these were funded by the eight regional health boards, while others were funded directly by the Department of Health. In addition, a range of voluntary agencies, particularly those for the elderly, disabled and children, receive all or part of their funding from the public system.

The sheer number, size and variation in the healthcare providers outlined above illustrate the extent of the challenge involved in deciding how much each agency should receive. The first major decision is taken by the Department of Health; the other major funders are the eight regional Health Boards which distribute their resources after they have received their own allocation from the Department. However, as noted above, the Department also funds some major agencies at local level, including public voluntary hospitals and homes for the mentally handicapped. Work is under way to transfer funding of these agencies to the health boards.[1]

The fact that the Department and, to an increasing extent, the Health Boards are major funders of publicly financed health services raises the question of how resources are actually allocated each year between so many competing providers. A number of key themes can be identified in the work on resource allocation decisions. These are:

- a conscious move away from incrementalist decision-making
- the development of more systematic decision-making tools for resource allocation, including case-mix budgeting in acute hospitals
- a growing emphasis on linking funding to agreed levels of service.

The departure from incrementalism

Traditionally, the budgets of publicly funded health agencies were heavily influenced by the money allocated in the previous year. Adjustments would then be made by reference to such factors as the total amount allocated to health services for the current year, agreed new developments, increased costs from pay awards, and service-specific items relevant to each agency.

The most serious disadvantage of this method of resource allocation is that it does not question the basis for the 'original' allocation; it merely offers marginal adjustments each year without reference to whether the agency's budget on establishment was itself 'correct' or reasonable. Few would argue that this approach to resource allocation is satisfactory, unless the basis for the original funding has been set using rigorous analysis of costs and activity. Even then, there is no guarantee that any subsequent incremental adjustments can successfully reflect genuine changes in costs or quality of service, as opposed to improvements in efficiency.

It is not easy to move away from incrementalist methods of resource allocation: they are more easily applied, offer greater predict-

---

[1] In November 1996 the Minister for Health announced that an Eastern Regional Health Authority would be established and would have responsibility for the funding of all health and personal social services in Dublin, Kildare and Wicklow. He also set up a high level Task Force to oversee and manage the implementation process and to work out the detailed organisational and administrative arrangements for the transition to the new structures. The Task Force submitted an Interim Report to the Minister in June 1997.

ability and involve less sudden change than more 'scientific' approaches. However, there is general acceptance that there must be greater emphasis on more objective indicators of funding requirements (see in particular the Health Strategy, *Shaping a Healthier Future* (1994)). The considerable improvements in data on health services in Ireland, particularly in the hospital area, permit closer analyses of the needs and performance of agencies. While this will not necessarily bring sudden or radical changes to the annual budgets of health agencies, it at least offers greater scope for a conscious move away from predominantly incrementalist decision-making.

Case-mix budgeting

The most tangible departure from incrementalist funding in Ireland has been the growing use of case-mix data to influence the resources allocated to acute hospitals. A case-mix budget model, in operation with continuing modification since 1993, is now used to measure the costs and activity of 30 acute public hospitals. Virtually all hospitals with more than 5,000 acute in-patient discharges are now covered. After differences in the complexity of caseload between hospitals are taken into account using recognised case-mix measures, the relative average costs per case can be judged more accurately. The case-mix budget model can then adjust each participating hospital's total allocation by reference to its case-mix-measured performance. An outline of how the case-mix budget operates is given in IPA fact sheets 5/94 and 6/94.

The case-mix budget model is *budget neutral*, in that it redistributes the existing funding available for acute hospitals. Some hospitals gain while others lose funding by reference to case-mix measures of costs and activity. This may at first seem to be primarily an incrementalist approach, since it merely moves some of the available funding between designated hospitals. However, the model is cumulative in its effect: the amounts gained or lost through case-mix are permanent adjustments to the hospital's baseline budget. Their cumulative effect over a period of some years can be substantial (Fitzgerald & Lynch, 1998). In any event, the performance of hospitals after five years of case-mix adjustments indicates that average costs are being pushed towards the centre: the signals sent by even modest case-mix adjustments have produced a noticeable convergence between hospitals of similar type.

While the case-mix budget model applies only to acute hospitals at present, the intention is to extend it over the next few years to maternity and paediatric hospitals as soon as the data sets in those hospitals permit. In the longer term, there seems little reason why the principles of case-mix in acute hospitals could not be applied to other sectors, such as mental health, mental handicap and community-based services. The critical requirement is a valid classification system for these patients and clients: in acute hospitals, classifications such as diagnosis related groups (DRGs) can be employed to group patients into meaningful categories based on clinical and financial indicators. Work is proceeding internationally to develop equivalent classification systems for other service areas.

Linking funding to activity

While case-mix funding is currently applicable only to the acute hospital sector, there are other methods of moving away from largely incrementalist methods of resource allocation. Increasingly, the emphasis is on relating the level of funding approved to agreed levels and types of service that must be provided. For example, the Health (Amendment) (No. 3) Act 1996 requires health boards to draw up a service plan consistent with the funds available to them. There is also a growing emphasis on providing for specific levels and types of service: this is evidenced by the recent *Waiting List Initiatives* in which hospitals were invited to tender for specific services (such as orthopaedic and ENT procedures) at a cost per case to be quoted by the hospital. Funds have then been allocated in return for a specified level of activity.

The ability of health boards to conclude service agreements with the agencies they fund is often hampered by data deficiencies, particularly where the detail of services provided by agencies is sketchy. However, it may be expected that the link between the amount of funds allocated and agreements on service levels will grow in the coming years.

Evaluation of services

Finally, a regular theme of recent commentaries on health spending internationally has been the importance of assessing not only the number and types of services provided but also the practical effect of those services. No longer is it acceptable merely to demonstrate that the money allocated to health and personal social services was spent *efficiently* on the areas for which it was intended; the emphasis is now switching to evaluating the *effectiveness* of the services provided. This is the critical distinction between *outputs*, such as number of services provided, number of clients seen or number of sessions worked, and *outcomes*, which are concerned with the actual result of the inter-vention.

Shaping a Healthier Future places particular emphasis on this issue, drawing attention to the concepts of *health gain* and *social gain*. Both concepts are used to underline the need for patients and clients to receive a clear benefit from their contact with the health system: health gain focuses on achieving improvements in health status, including increases in life expectancy and cure or alleviation of illness or disability, while social gain is concerned with adding quality to life, particularly in the context of longer-term services such as those for the elderly or children at risk. Evaluating outcomes of health services is a very difficult task; it asks some difficult questions about whether (and to what extent) the provision of a service made a positive difference to the life or well-being of patients and clients. Techniques for this form of evaluation are still in their infancy, but they address the type of questions that health services in all countries must seek to answer to ensure that finite health expenditure is allocated to services that truly improve the health or well-being of patients, clients and their families. At a time when sometimes simplistic questions are asked about whether 'enough money' is being spent on healthcare, it is perhaps well to remember that the major issue for the future is what we are achieving with the available resources.

CHAPTER 7

Resource Management in the Irish and UK Health Systems – Reconciling the Irreconcilable?

Marie Brady and Peter West

Introduction

Health systems throughout the Western world are struggling to reconcile ever-increasing demand for acute hospital services with the resources available. Ireland and the UK are no exceptions, though they have adopted different approaches to coping with the challenge. The need for resource management at hospital level is the focus of this chapter.

The chapter identifies the main approaches to resource management adopted in Ireland and the UK. It starts with the premise that there are pressures in both systems that can result in non-rational allocation of resources. Chief among these is the system of fixed budgets, but variable (usually additional) demand. Others stem from the intrinsically unplannable nature of hospital work, and some are to do with the nature of clinical autonomy. Having discussed the respective approaches, the chapter concludes that what is required is

- greater clarity as to what patients can expect from the hospital system, and clear protocols and guidelines for the treatments they receive, possibly through the service planning process in the Irish system
- the continuing involvement of clinicians at hospital level to provide input to the strategic and service/business planning processes, and to contribute to the day-to-day management of services.

The challenges that arise for health managers and policy-makers include

- getting the issue of 'what treatment for what patients' onto the health policy agenda
- creating and maintaining the right conditions for clinicians to become more involved in hospital leadership and management
- ensuring effective processes of hospital service planning that have the active involvement and commitment of resource users, especially doctors.

Issues in resource management

The healthcare systems of Ireland and the UK have many similarities, as well as some fundamental differences. Both have strong traditions of relatively independent GPs, but with substantial differences in the way that they are paid. Both have salaried hospital doctors but with differences in the proportion of private fee-paying patients. Both systems have funded hospitals through block grants in the past, with allocations based on historic funding and annual adjustments, but in recent years they have differed appreciably in the funding mechanisms. The UK NHS introduced an internal market, and recent Labour proposals will continue to keep purchasers and providers separate. Ireland has introduced elements of activity funding for hospitals, based on DRGs.

Both systems have tended to limit the resources going to a hospital, through block grant and contract funding, and both systems have limits on expenditure which mean that increased activity by hospitals will not necessarily lead to increased income. The underlying features of resource management are increasingly shared by hospitals in other countries as health systems have increasingly moved away from fee-for-service medicine in which costs are reimbursed for individual patients. Managed care in all its manifestations increasingly means that the resources available to treat a given group of patients are constrained and the clinical decisions of those treating the patients must be reconciled with the funding decisions of those paying for care, through public or private insurance.

Squaring the circle – fixed funds and variable demand

Much of what follows on the specific details of resource management in UK and Irish hospitals is conditioned by the fundamental funding issue that confronts hospital doctors and others responsible for prescribing the pattern of care for patients. If the funding for a hospital and an individual speciality or department is fixed, by whatever means, then the uncertainties of medical demands will lead to overspending (or potentially underspending) from time to time. The balance between emergency and non-emergency patients will change, new treatments will become available, patients will differ in their social and domestic circumstances and will require different lengths of stay and periods of rehabilitation. While these might average out over a number of years, two other aspects of tight funding make life difficult for clinicians. First, it is often difficult to carry forward savings from years of lower demand to years of higher demand. Second, there are often internal advantages in using resources when demand is lower, to enhance patient care or protect departmental resources. For example, a period of low demand for emergency surgery or trauma can only be determined retrospectively. As a result, surgeons enjoying lower demands may prefer to treat additional waiting list cases rather than transferring beds or other resources to physicians. Loss of beds to medical cases may be difficult to recoup if demand suddenly increases, and so a quiet year for emergency surgery need not translate into a low-spending year for surgical services.

A related difficulty is that if technology changes rapidly in a clinical area, the overall level of health funding may not change as fast. Even if annual growth in funding is sufficient, in aggregate, to meet the costs of new technologies in the limited number of departments where a significant technical change has occurred, it may be difficult within hospitals to allocate a disproportionate share of growth to one department. Every department will be able to show some need for additional resources at the margin, to reduce waiting lists or improve the quality of care, even in the absence of technical change. As a result, doctors in many departments will at any time see themselves in serious competition for funds with their colleagues rather than as sharing in a clearly planned and rational allocation. The use of a variety of non-rational allocation methods inside hospitals may result from the imposition of so many tensions on the organisation through tight external funding.

Resource management in the UK National Health Service

Since 1991, the NHS has operated an internal market. While this will change as a result of proposals from the Labour government, it seems likely that an element of separation between those buying or commissioning services and those providing them will continue. District Health Authorities with populations of about 500,000 or more currently purchase under contract from NHS Trust hospitals and community care providers. GP fund-holders separately hold budgets for non-emergency care. In future, groups of up to 50 GPs will lead purchasing of all services for populations of up to 100,000.

Contracts are of various kinds and specify costs and volumes of patients to be treated. Some contracts may be closer to a block model, in which a service is commissioned for an unspecified number of patients but with a fixed capacity or some other limit on expenditure. This kind of contract can shift some of the risk of fluctuating demands for treatment from the purchasers to the providers. However, if the capacity is not sufficient and additional expenditure is needed to cope (actually or allegedly), then the purchasers may none the less have to meet the demand. For example, the demands for emergency hospital treatment have risen in the UK in recent years and forced many health authorities to overspend on contracts.

In elective surgery, there is much more scope for specifying costs, volumes and other factors, such as the extent to which patients are treated as day cases. However, there are some limitations on contracts even in this area. Two difficulties in particular have tended to dominate contracting and pricing.

Firstly, although the NHS has improved its data collection dramatically in recent years, this is not yet in a state where a detailed account of patients can be compiled in a way which is necessary for resource management. Diagnostic codes, for example, may give no indication of severity. Procedure codes may not indicate whether a patient is undergoing a procedure for the first time or having a revision and even where additional codes exist, these may not be well used by clinicians. Other factors, e.g. home circumstances, which may affect discharge decisions, are simply not recorded on routine hospital records and so an incomplete set of information is available on which to base pricing in contracts. The simplest solution would be to refine the data collection in each department, concentrating initially on the procedures or diagnoses which make up the greatest part of the total cost. However, instituting additional local data collection is not popular and so a satisfactory picture of local activity may not be available.

For example, a purchaser of a surgical procedure should ideally know:

- the number of patients referred for assessment with a query diagnosis
- the proportion of these patients undergoing each subsequent diagnostic test, especially relatively costly imaging procedures and invasive tests such as endoscopy and angiography
- the proportion of patients progressing to surgery
- the length of stay and resource use of surgical patients
- the reasons for outliers and year-on-year variance in cost per case
- the outcome in health gain.

Given all these data, the purchaser can begin to develop a rolling plan for this type of surgery and make financial provision for it. But in practice purchasers lack both the data linkages and the human resources to develop their contract planning in this degree of detail.

The second difficulty is that pricing is still in its infancy in the NHS and, because contracting has mainly been handled locally and not nationally, there are wide discrepancies in prices between providers for similar procedures. US healthcare agencies such as Medicare typically set prices for particular procedures and impose these across their many providers. While there is bound to be an element of arbitrariness in any price for a hospital case (because the overhead costs of the hospital can be apportioned to each case in several different ways), a fixed price ensures consistency. Local price variation in the NHS means that the connection between activities and resources is neither constant nor accurate, and so any resource plans within hospitals that are linked to contract income may be flawed.

Before examining how resources are managed within hospitals, we should note that any system which has a cash limit on total spending is bound to have some difficulties in managing resources once these become part of a contract that rewards activity. One tool of managed care in many systems is to press a capitation contract onto providers, asking them to provide services for a defined population for a fixed fee, so that activity does not affect expenditure for the purchaser. The provider has to bear the risks of fluctuations in the demands of the population. This approach is much more likely to succeed, however, where a provider has access to a range of services for patients at different costs. Hence the enthusiasm of total fund-holding GP practices. They can offer patients a package of hospital, GP and community nurse/therapist care which can make sure that all patients receive a service but which limits the number of patients receiving hospital care. In contrast, a hospital-only provider, denied the opportunity to provide family and community care by the current NHS rules and regulations of the market, can only treat patients in its own high-cost facilities. It has one mode of response and will find it more difficult to manage fluctuating demands within the capitation payment.

In consequence, the cash-limited system with fluctuating demands on it will, from time to time, generate considerable tension between the costs of treating additional patients, the rewards for doing so and the lack of funds to do so. Compared to a conventional market, where volume is linked to income, this tension may be a cause of considerable frustration. Even if it is possible that the tension could be removed by greater efficiency by providers, as some have argued, this does not solve the problem that individual units and departments may from time to time feel the stress of rising demands without being confident that they will enjoy the rewards of extra activity.

Resource management in the Irish public hospital system

The Irish health system has adopted a variety of approaches to resource management in acute hospitals. As in the UK, hospitals were funded on an incremental block-grant system. A system of direct funding from the DOH meant that voluntary hospitals, which provide much of the service in the Eastern region and other major centres, had no formal accountability to their regional Health Boards. Since 1993, the DOH has incorporated a case-mix adjustment within the resource allocation process in acute hospitals, beginning with the larger hospitals but now almost countrywide. The proportion of the budget calculated on this basis has increased from 5% to 15%, and may be increased in future.

This approach resulted in significant reductions and additions in resources for the hospitals involved in the first two years, but most have now adjusted towards the mean. This is partly due to hospitals supplying more comprehensive data for case-mix calculation. The DOH sees the potential of DRGs as a common language for clinicians and policy-makers, especially in relation to service outcomes and service planning. The Health (Amendment) (No. 3) Act 1996, which was expected to come into force early in 1998, will have a significant impact on resource management. The Act clarifies the respective roles of Health Boards and their Chief Executives. It requires each board to develop an annual service plan, along explicit lines, and to involve health professionals in the process. It also provides that any excess in spending in one year is carried over as a first charge on the following year's income. The restructuring of the Eastern Health Board area will also have a significant impact, and is expected to come into force beginning in 1999. The region will be managed by a Regional Council and three Area Councils. Voluntary agencies across the entire system will no longer be funded directly from the DOH, but by each regional Health Board. This should provide for a more coherent approach to service planning and resource management.

Resource management within NHS hospitals

Within NHS hospitals, the most common mechanism for resource management is the clinical directorate. This structure has emerged in part because of a growing recognition that if the clinicians, as the key actors determining the use of resources, are not heavily involved in managing activities then the activities are not likely to be well managed by others. Medicine has a culture of independence and equality among consultant staff, in part the result of a lack of evidence on the right way to treat many conditions, and hospital consultants are likely to adopt their own policies in treating patients. Clinical directors – consultant staff appointed to manage the directorate with and through their colleagues – are more likely to be accepted as managers of doctors than professional managers or accountants.

The thrust towards clinical directorates was given much greater emphasis after the 1993 Griffiths Report on the management of the NHS, but the ideas behind it had been around for a considerable time before that. Griffiths was concerned that in many areas of hospital activity it was not clear who was in charge, and argued for a general manager or chief executive who would take ultimate responsibility. This system replaced the previous consensus models in 1984 and was reinforced by the move to Trust status after 1991, which gave hospitals a (nominally) increased degree of independence, making NHS hospitals somewhat similar to voluntary hospitals in Ireland, no longer under direct management by a health authority.

Clinical directorates were part of a 'chain of command' from the Chief Executive, via the Board of Directors, to each clinical department or speciality. The Board of Directors would typically include clinical directors and directors of finance, personnel and nursing, though the precise structure was left to individual trusts to resolve. Larger hospitals, such as the major teaching hospitals, typically have groups of directorates (e.g. surgery, medicine, women and children) represented at Board level and separate directorates at the next level down.

Although clinical directorates were introduced to lead their departments and improve resource management, it is important to note the differences between this role and a similar role in the private sector. To a degree, management is consensual in all organisations. If employees do not agree with management policy, they may not carry it out or may carry it out weakly or ineffectively. The greater the management's power to discipline or replace disaffected workers, the easier it is to ensure that management decisions are followed. But even the strictest private-sector firm cannot shoot staff for desertion, and managerial bullies like the late Robert Maxwell are probably rare! Sackings and disciplinings bring their own counterblasts in strikes and bad publicity and so a consensus of some kind is always the likely outcome of management decisions, though the extent to which the consensus reflects the aims of management or staff will vary with the degree of power management can exert.

Once a decision is reached, however, the key feature of line management is that it is clear where the responsibility lies. Management has insisted on a policy and management will take the consequences. In clinical work, and other professional services, this poses a difficulty. The individual doctor has a duty and responsibility to the patient to provide appropriate treatment. 'Appropriate' is relatively poorly defined, and while it remains so there is a tension between doing what is best for patients, as judged by the clinician, and doing what management requires. This difficulty is exacerbated by the relative flatness of the top of the clinical hierarchy. Consultants are likely to see themselves as equal, and may refuse to accept the authority of their clinical director in some aspects of their work. As a result, the clinical directorate may show a wide range of treatments and policies, the best compromise that the clinical director can achieve. Because clinical directors are usually appointed from within the existing consultants, and often rotate after a number of terms, they may not always have the necessary skills and personalities for effective management. So we should not be surprised to find that clinical directorates do not solve all the problems of managing resources. Rather, they provide a framework within which resource management issues can be taken forward, and solved in at least a proportion of cases. Where the clinical director commands the professional respect of colleagues and has the right personality and skills for effective management, clinical directorates can be particularly effective.

Resource management at directorate level

The typical clinical directorate has a business manager who obtains financial and activity information from the trust and uses it with the clinical director to plan and monitor the work of the directorate. A directorate plan may include information on:

- patient numbers, perhaps by major diagnosis or procedure, as determined by contract negotiations with purchasers
- available resources, including wards and bed days
- targets for the use of resources, e.g. average length of patient stay, extent of day case surgery
- budgets and forecasts for drug expenditure and use of other departments' resources, e.g. diagnostic testing.

Routine monthly monitoring will then indicate how far planned activity and expenditure are being achieved and what, if any, variances are occurring. The major causes of variance are likely to be examined and resolved either by internal agreement or by referral upwards. For example, a rising number of emergency admissions might be met by reviewing admissions policies and ensuring that senior staff are involved in the assessment of borderline cases, and by requesting that trust management review the contract for emergency admissions with purchasers to bring contracted activity up towards the actual level achieved. Rising drug expenditure might be examined by reviewing drug policy internally but also by asking for additional resources when new and more expensive drugs become available.

Resource management at Irish hospital level

Doctors have always been involved in hospital decision-making structures, through membership of Medical Boards, Medical Councils, Medical Executives, etc. and through membership of Hospital

Advisory Committees, Hospital Management Committees, etc. with Directors of Nursing and Hospital Administrators. In the past, Irish consultants shared the general reluctance to become more involved in hospital management, because of

- the heavy time commitment involved which would cut into other activities
- a perception that they lacked some of the necessary skills, especially financial ones
- a lack of well-developed information systems
- a concern about how their peers would accept them in a managerial context.

The consultants' contract of 1991 provided for the development of practice plans by individual consultants. It also provided for clinical co-ordinators, to co-ordinate the integration of practice plans into a coherent pattern of service provision for the coming year. It was decided not to adopt the clinical directorate model generally, but to pilot different structures and systems appropriate to individual hospitals and Health Boards.

The development of individual practice plans never really got off the ground, partly because of the absence of adequate information systems to support them in the early stages, and partly because of budgetary constraints and the priority on cost containment. Clinical co-ordinators were appointed in some, but not all, hospitals. The new consultants' contract is likely to provide for a more direct role for consultants in hospital management, and also for a key role for consultant involvement in service planning at speciality, rather than individual consultant, level. Pilot schemes of clinical directorates, hospital policy teams, etc. have been in operation for some time, and some are now well established. Other hospitals have begun to follow suit with their own customised versions, based mostly on the clinical directorate model. An alternative strategy adopted by some Health Boards has been to strengthen the general management and information support systems in anticipation of formal management structures involving consultants.

Conclusions

Clinical directorates (and other approaches) cannot resolve all the problems of resource management in hospitals. As long as health systems fail to specify what treatment should be provided for what patients, there will always be considerable and legitimate scope for clinical discretion. High-spending doctors may well be doing their best for patients and may not be inefficient. Low-spending doctors may be providing too little care and not merely being parsimonious with public money. In the absence of clear protocols and guidelines for treatment in purchasers' contracts, this kind of variation may be inevitable. But that does not eliminate the advantages of resource management through clinical directorates.

In the last analysis, unplanned use of resources in hospitals which have a limited budget must impact on patients and their clinicians. While it is easy to sympathise with clinicians who seek autonomy in the best interests of their patients, if all the consultants in a hospital operate with the maximum degree of autonomy they are likely to come into conflict with each other over resource use. By developing consistent plans for activities and resources, albeit plans which will not be met fully or exactly, the clinical directorate structure can reduce the scope for conflicting demands on resources. Where conflicts due to autonomous resource use cannot be resolved, the fact that there has been an explicit debate about them will at least allow better planning of the consequences. Resource management through clinical directorates is not a recipe for complete consistency or stable planning, but it has clear advantages over the anarchy of independent clinical practice.

This analysis raises several challenges for health service managers and policy-makers. The first two are particularly relevant – though not exclusively so – to the Irish context; the third is common to both systems and, indeed, to public health systems generally. The challenges are:

- to create and maintain the right conditions for clinicians to become involved effectively in hospital leadership and management – medical involvement is a lynchpin in effective resource management
- to make a realistic assessment of the time commitment required by clinicians to perform these leadership and management roles effectively
- to design structures that are appropriate to individual hospitals or health boards – hospitals vary enormously in terms of size, nature of service provided, organisational culture, etc.; no single

model is likely to meet the needs of all hospitals

- to enable clinicians in managerial roles to network with colleagues in similar roles, to identify role models and provide peer support
- to provide training and development in the skills and competencies required for the managerial role, especially clinical leadership skills
- to develop and maintain effective relationships and mutual respect between consultants, nursing and general management
- to ensure effective processes of hospital service planning that have the active involvement and commitment of resource users, especially doctors – this will be facilitated by using a multi-disciplinary approach to both planning and service evaluation, supported by information systems at clinical and service activity levels.

PART FOUR

Changing Management Practice

CHAPTER 8

Balancing Risk-taking and Accountability in Public-Sector Management

DENIS DOHERTY

Introduction

> Risk is inherent in a commitment of present resources to future expectations. Indeed economic progress can be defined as the ability to take greater risks. The attempt to eliminate risks, even the attempt to minimise them, can only make them irrational and unbearable. It can only result in the greatest risk of all; rigidity. (Drucker, 1973)

My first promotion, nearly 30 years ago, was to the position of Town Clerk, Midleton. My new job was very different to the previous one of Clerical Officer in the Accounts Department of Donegal County Council. The County Manager invited me to meet with him at his office on the morning I took up my new position. Our meeting was brief, but the advice he gave me was inspiring. He reminded me that Town Clerks of Midleton got promoted quickly, and said 'You'll be remembered for what you do for the town, and I won't be impressed if the feedback I get is that you are doing a good job in the office'. Michael Conlon was an enlightened and progressive County Manager who instilled confidence and enthusiasm in those who worked for him. In the year I spent in Midleton I learned a great deal from his style and approach to public service management. My experience of having worked in an accounts department was to stand to me during that year also. I spotted a financial irregularity, at a sufficiently early stage to avoid it causing a serious financial loss to the Council or blighting the career of the Town Clerk! The lesson I took from that experience is that public service management should seek to achieve a balance between the need to be accountable to the public for the way their money is spent, and a prudent degree of risk-taking in the interests of producing a better service.

A theme of this chapter, therefore, is that of achieving balance. This recurs in discussion of public v. private, citizen v. customer, risk v. accountability, and in relation to the potential of wealth-generating organisations, business organisations and service organisations to shape collectively the communities of the future by recognising how interdependent they are and how achieving the correct balance will influence them for the better. The concepts of investing for social return and managing for social result are put forward as the public-sector equivalents of investing for financial return and managing for financial return in the private sector.

Balancing public versus private sector

Public-sector managers are often exhorted to behave more like their private-sector counterparts, who are portrayed as more entre-preneurial, customer-responsive and bottom-line-focused. Based on similar thinking, the public sector is exhorted to become more like business. Mintzberg (1996) disputes the claim that government must become more like business, and argues that 'if we are to manage government properly, then we must learn to govern management'. Mintzberg argues in favour of balance between the public and private sectors. He holds the view that in the West we have been living in balanced societies with strong private sectors, strong public sectors, and great strength in the sectors in between. He attributes the failure of communist regimes to the fact that they got totally out of balance.

Citizens are, of course, entitled to expect that public-sector organisations will operate efficiently, effectively and with an emphasis on quality improvement, value for money, and so on. In those respects there are more similarities than differences between the public and private sectors. Public- and private-sector organisations both tend to be controlled by hierarchical structures. Private and commercial organisations, though, are much easier to understand than their public-sector counterparts. They exist to achieve financial return on investments through the generation of profits. Until relatively recently, most private and commercial organisations did not see themselves as having social obligations. Concerns about issues like environmental damage caused by industrial pollution, use of animals for researching consumer products, and accessibility of premises to persons with disabilities have caused many private-sector organisations to reconsider their social obligations. Some concerns which were initially articulated by pressure groups and dismissed as of interest only to minorities have in time won wide public support. Many private-sector organisations have come to accept that they are accountable to citizens and communities as well as to their shareholders.

Managing for social result

It is more difficult to understand the *raison d'être* of many public service organisations, and in trying to do so I have found it helpful to seek comparisons with the private sector. In the case of the health services, for example, the taxpayer is the investor, but has no choice other than to invest, for the purpose of achieving a social return in the form of the healthcare standards citizens can aspire to as a result of that investment. Until recently, accountability in terms of activity, size of waiting lists, absence of waste and such was accepted. But now, accountability in the form of measurable returns is expected. Managers in the public service must, therefore, manage for social results in the way that managers in the commercial sector manage for financial results. Public-sector organisations must address the bottom line of social return on investment in the way that commercial organisations address their bottom line of financial return on investment. It is very much easier to measure financial results and financial returns than it is to measure social results and social returns. The justification for taking calculated risks in the public sector must, none the less, be the social return that will accrue if the risk is overcome.

There remains the difficulty of demonstrating social return. It often appears that the absence of a financial bottom line results in public-sector organisations being less objectively and more harshly judged than their private-sector counterparts. Savoie (1995) comments that

> in business, it does not much matter if you get it wrong 10% of the time as long as you turn in a profit at the end of the year. In government, it does not much matter if you get it right 90% of the time because the focus will be on the 10% of the time you get it wrong.

The child protection experience I refer to later would tend to bear out that view.

Citizen versus customer

Exhortations to the public service to become more like business are often less than fully thought through. Customers of the public service are primarily citizens of the state. The adage 'let the buyer beware' instils a certain cautionary approach in customers dealing with business, but citizens dealing with an agency of the state expect the state to protect their interests.

When adapted to Irish circumstances, an illustration used by Tom Peters in one of his newsletters points up the dichotomy that can arise between citizens and customers.

> If I apply to the planning authority for permission to extend my home, I am unlikely to object if they view me as their customer. But if my next door neighbour applies to extend his home and I am opposed to the proposal, who now is the customer of the planning authority?

The answer of course is that when a citizen deals with an agency of the state, the relationship is not that of a willing seller and a willing buyer but that of a citizen accessing a legal entitlement and being liable to the constraints involved in being a subject of the state. Organisations providing social services have a duty and an obligation to demonstrate goodness of their product. It is essential not that the service be without risk, but that it be delivered fairly and equitably. The small risk associated with the administration of some vaccines, for example, is considered to be justified by the greater good accruing to society at large from the prevention of communicable disease afforded by successful vaccination programmes. The challenge is to strike an acceptable balance between the rights of individual citizens and the common good.

Risk management

The term 'risk management' is used in this chapter to describe the entrepreneurial aspect of public management rather than the health and safety context in which that term is also used. The Virtues English Dictionary definition of risk as 'to venture or to dare to undertake' seems particularly suited to the context in which it is used here.

Arising from the developing interest in risk-taking in public-

service management among academics and public service practitioners in the UK, Jeremy Vincent (1996) carried out a review of the
international literature on the subject on behalf of the Centre for
Public Services Management, London. He found that the literature
reflects governance and accountability issues rather than risk
management. Questions of risk are implied and alluded to in different
ways, but one gets the impression that the question of risk management, as an important topic in its own right, is not yet deemed suitable
for open debate. The tentative approach to risk management is well
illustrated in an American context by Bryson (1988), who comments
that:

> The public sector is a particularly hard place for people to take risks – and
> therefore learn without punishment

and goes on to recommend that

> public organisations and their employees must systematically make enough
> small mistakes so that they can learn but not enough so that they are
> punished.

The problem with that attitude is that risk-taking and entrepreneurship
get practised only at the margins. Value is added when managers are
trained how to calculate risks accurately and supported in the decisions
they take, based on their judgement of the benefits that will result
from succeeding over the risks associated with failing. Risk-taking is
more likely to succeed when encouraged in a context in which the
goals of the organisation are clear. Strategic planning and strategic
management involve adopting strategies, i.e. the means through which
the goals of the organisation become performance. The adoption of
strategies involves, in turn, the calculation and judgement of the risks
involved. 'Risk management recognises that mistakes will be made
but should not be repeatedly made' (Management Advisory Board,
1993). The Management Advisory Board (1993) in Australia takes
the view that 'adoption of a risk management approach has not led
to any diminution in the requirement for due process, but rather to
a heightened focus on cost effective outcomes'.

Irish solutions to an international dilemma

In Ireland the Comptroller and Auditor General (Amendment) Act
1993 and the Strategic Management Initiative in the public sector

created the climate in which the balance between accountability and risk management will develop and be judged. John Hurley (Secretary, Public Service Management and Development, Department of Finance) (1995) summarised strategic management in the civil service in Ireland as follows.

> In essence, it is a process designed to place more focus on likely future developments thus enabling a more effective and informed response to be made to the challenges ahead. The underlying approach is geared to ensuring a critical self examination of what we are doing, why we are doing it and how well we are performing. It is also designed, therefore, to make us more result oriented and to get the best out of the available resources. A key outcome should be improved services to the public.

On the subject of accountability and responsibility, Hurley (1995) had this to say:

> Accountability should affect everything we do. In practice, though, it is normally concerned only with the big issues, and then mainly in a financial context. But accountability in the true sense should extend to a complete appraisal of our responsibilities and performance, the effectiveness of our actions and our contribution to the organisation as a whole, and in the final analysis the extent to which the citizen and taxpayer have received the best possible services and value for money. Our existing framework of accountability – through the Ministers and Secretaries Acts – has been with us since the foundation of the state and it is timely to review it, in the light of today's more complex and fast changing environment. Many would argue that the framework impedes flexibility and hampers the effective devolution of responsibility and accountability.

Civil servants propose risk-tolerant culture

Government departments and state agencies are individually responding to the Strategic Management Initiative, and in addition a group of Secretaries of Government Departments is co-ordinating the work. The Second Report to Government of this Co-ordinating Group of Secretaries (*Delivering Better Government*, 1996) stated that

> it has long been recognised that the existing structures and reporting systems promote a risk averse environment where taking personal responsibility is not encouraged and, equally, where innovative approaches to service delivery have not been developed... The Group believe that

legislative change is required, in particular, to clarify the allocation of authority, accountability and responsibility in the system... It may be said that many departments view existing expenditure controls as over centralised, heavy handed and short-term in orientation... The Group recommend that, in keeping with the increased emphasis on devolving responsibility and accountability, a more appropriate public financial framework for settling public expenditure allocations, and delegating authority to departments to manage resources allocated to them, be put in place.

The transition from a 'risk-averse' environment to a 'risk-tolerant' one represents a truly mammoth task, which involves much more than just changing the public service. It involves securing the approval of the citizenry and the body politic. It involves achieving balance between the expectations and the entitlements of citizens from their public service. It should mean that public servants will be judged on the results they achieve and be given discretion in relation to the means they employ to achieve the results expected of them.

Pilot projects

The Report of the Co-Ordinating Group of Secretaries identifies the following seven issues to be assigned to cross-departmental teams to be co-ordinated by a Minister/Minister of State and with a specific lead department:

- child-care
- drugs
- employment
- competitiveness
- unemployment and social exclusion
- financial services
- local development.

Interestingly, the recommendation goes on to state unambiguously that 'a clear obligation would be placed on the team to develop solutions and new approaches. Suitable reward mechanisms will need to be designed for this work.' This approach is interesting for a number of reasons. The emphasis on developing solutions and new approaches implies acceptance that new ways of doing things will be needed and, by extension, that risks not encountered before will be experienced.

The recognition that reward mechanisms will be needed is significant. Failure is not contemplated, at least not in terms of recommending sanctions if solutions or new approaches are not found. However, failure to reap the incentives on offer could be viewed as a form of sanction which would not have the negative connotations of the formal imposition of penalties. The list of issues chosen is also interesting for the reason that accountability considerations will be much broader than merely giving account that the money involved was properly spent and that value for money was achieved. It is obvious that managers are being encouraged to manage strategically and that measurable achievement of strategic goals will be the basis for judgement.

Achieving a social return on investment

Child protection – choosing the lesser of two risks

The choice of child-care as an issue is of particular interest to me – it is a subject that I have spoken on and written about (Doherty, 1996). Up to relatively recently it was considered that the interests of children at serious risk were best satisfied by taking them into care. There was a belief that residential child-care was of a uniformly high standard and that all those involved in caring for children observed the trust placed in them. While that was generally true, we now know that for many children placement in care resulted in their being abused by those to whose care they were entrusted. I take the view that the constant flow of child-abuse scandals of recent years has challenged the very core of our perceptions of ourselves as a people and that we are experiencing enormous difficulty, as a nation, in coming to terms with the pervasiveness of this problem. In Doherty (1996) I stated that

> I have concerns regarding our collective reaction to these events and in particular to the evolving negative attitude to service providers in the child protection field. Rather than developing a balanced picture which recognises the enormous complexity of the child protection task and the commitment and professionalism of current service providers, we are entering into judgements based on limited understanding. Increasing numbers of staff are, sadly, coming to view child protection work as thankless and professionally risky.

A decision to remove a child from its natural family is an onerous one and should arise only when it is judged that the risk of not removing the child is greater than the risk and disadvantages associated with placing the child in an alternative setting. Learning, leading to best practice, is achieved through experience based on experimentation. We need to distinguish between abuse of trust and reckless behaviour, on the one hand, and calculated risk-taking and well-intentioned experimentation, aimed at improving learning and best practice, on the other. The choice in child protection is often a matter of choosing the lesser of two risks. We are a long way from being able to measure social return from investment in the protection of children.

In Doherty (1996), I posed a number of questions:

> I wonder if our desire to establish the facts of what occurred in the past is contributing, in the way we hope it is, to learning, leading to improvements in current child-care practices and thereby reducing the risk that the present generation of children in care will grow up with bad memories of their time in care?... Is there a danger that by dwelling on past failures we will fail to do sufficient to match current practice to the care needs of this generation of children who need care and protection from the state?

I went on to advocate that

> Our efforts as policy-makers and managers must recognise that the success of our child-care services passes unnoticed by those not directly involved, while failures and mistakes, however small their number may be relative to the total number of cases, are judged very severely indeed. That recognition must include providing support and welfare services to staff, whose work is of a stressful nature. The pursuit of higher standards may involve some mishaps on route. Staff must not be discouraged from taking calculated risks, they judge to be in the best interests of children, even if occasionally they get it wrong.

Moving and removing fences

Some years ago I was advised, by someone opposed to the pace of reform of our mental health services, that in rural Ireland there is a saying that 'one should not remove the fence without finding out why it was put there in the first place'. Looked at another way, a fence is an intrusion in the landscape, however strong the justification for it may be. As circumstances change the fence should be repositioned, and when the reasons which justified its erection in the first place no longer exist, it should be removed.

The mental health services in Ireland are an example of fences being kept in place for longer than they were needed. Improvements in treatment regimes and drug therapies justified their removal years earlier. The available research (e.g. Fitzpatrick *et al.*, 1995) suggests that the community-based approach to delivering services to the mentally ill is an improvement on the former hospital-based approach and justifies the perceived risks associated with such a fundamental change in the way an essential service is organised and delivered. Mental hospitals traditionally contained large numbers of patients inexpensively. The quality of life in supported hostels is judged to be superior for the residents and represents higher social return on the investment by society in a group of people previously highly marginalised by virtue of the illness they suffered from. Patients are unequivocal in their judgement of the value to them of the new arrangements. The social return to society is the value society places on the judgements arrived at by the recipients, on whose behalf that social investment is made. Some fences are still required – the Central Mental Hospital is an example of one. On the other hand, prison regimes are changing through the repositioning of fences.

Problems in measuring social result

The difficulty involved in measuring social result is encountered in many situations. Even within particular sectors, degrees of difficulty are involved. In the case of hospital surgical services, it is easier to measure outcomes in cataract removal surgery than in hip replacement surgery. In both cases considerations of, for example, recovery times, infection rates and complication rates are relevant. However, the most meaningful outcomes for the patients concerned are the extent to which they recover their sight in the case of cataract removal surgery, and reduction of pain and restored mobility in the case of hip replacement surgery. Objective measurement of eyesight recovery is possible, but measurement of pain reduction and mobility improvement is much more subjective. Mintzberg (1996) illustrates the difficulty of measuring outcomes in surgery with the following example.

> A liver transplant surgeon in the national health service operated on ten patients. Two died. Of the eight who survived, one who had cancer years

earlier suffered a recurrence. Another patient's liver began to fail and he needed a second transplant. Of the remaining six patients only three were able to resume normal working lives. Asked about his performance, the surgeon claimed his success rate as eight in ten. (Indeed, as soon as he replaced the failing liver, he was prepared to claim nine in eleven. He counted livers, not people.) An immunologist put it at seven in ten, believing that the surgeon should not have operated on the person who had had cancer. A cost conscious Hospital Administrator put the figure at six in ten. The nurses claimed three in ten, taking into account post-operative quality of life.

Mintzberg used this example to illustrate his view that many areas of the public service don't lend themselves to precise measurement and that assessment of many of the most common activities in government require soft judgement – something that hard measurement cannot provide.

Advances in medical knowledge and technology are resulting in healthcare services developing a capacity to consume infinite amounts of resources. The argument is no longer about the need for rationing but about what criteria should be used in rationing and who should interpret the criteria. In the case of liver transplants, who should decide whether or not there should be a programme? Where it is decided to have a programme, how should the allocation of financial resources be determined? Where rationing is involved, what steps can be taken to achieve the desired balance between the nine-in-eleven success rating of the surgeon, on technical grounds, and the three-in-ten rating of the nurses, on quality of life grounds? In accountability terms, how can the social return from investment in a liver transplant programme best be measured in relation to other investment options? Is it possible at all to assess accurately and compare the option of investing in a liver transplant programme with the option of developing a community mental health service?

Accountability

If the issue of risk-taking has not received much explicit attention in Ireland and internationally, the issue of accountability has. There is no generally accepted definition of the term, though most definitions tend to incorporate the concept of being answerable to a superior for one's action. References to accountability in the public sector tend to couple the term 'responsibility' with it. Caiden (1988) describes these terms as follows.

> To be responsible is to have the authority to act, power to control, freedom to decide, the ability to distinguish (as between right and wrong) and to behave rationally and reliably and with consistency and trustworthiness in exercising internal judgement. To be accountable is to answer for one's responsibilities, to report, to explain, to give reasons, to respond, to assume obligations, to render a reckoning and submit to an outside or external judgement.

Kernaghan and Langford (1990) observe that

> Public servants are often accountable in several directions at once and can, therefore, receive conflicting signals as to what is expected of them.

In public-sector organisations in Ireland, that range of accountability can include some, or even all, of the following:

- to a superior
- to elected members
- to a government department
- to the Comptroller and Auditor General
- to the law
- to the Courts and the Ombudsman
- to social partners in respect of collective agreements
- to public-service ethos

and, of course

- to the public.

Accountability to the public is less formal and less structured than most of the others, but in practice public servants, especially those imbued with a strong sense of public service, take very seriously indeed their responsibilities to the public they serve. Admirable though this is, it can give rise to significant difficulties in practice. For example, it is understandable that doctors and nurses feel a strong sense of obligation to their patients which, in extreme situations, can take precedence over their sense of duty to their employers. This can give rise to controversy where decisions of that type result in financial budgets being exceeded. Most patients are also taxpayers, and the hospital that employs the doctors and nurses is accountable not just for the way it spent public money but also for ensuring that the amount of money entrusted to it was not exceeded. Once again the need to achieve balance between conflicting pressures arises.

Balancing accountability and risk-taking

There are some who hold the view that asking public officials to behave creatively and strategically on the one hand, and to be accountable to a multitude of constituencies on the other, is unrealistic and impossible. Gagne (1996) expresses this view as follows.

> Politicians and the public cannot have it both ways. They must choose whether they wish to have public servants become productivity and efficiency conscious or to have them remain essentially concerned with due process and fairness in their dealings with the public. If it is to be the former, then public servants must not only be accountable for their actions, they must also be given both the authority and the freedom to make administrative decisions commensurate with the degree of accountability thrust upon them. In like manner, public servants accorded greater authority and freedom to make administrative decisions must accept the risks associated with that authority, and they cannot expect elected officials to shoulder the blame when decisions go awry.

Wright (1996) disputes that point of view, and claims that

> While managerialist initiatives have increased the emphasis on efficiency and service at some possible expense to fairness and due process, the reality (as opposed to some of the rhetoric) has been one of finding a new balance that can accommodate the current fiscal reality and demands for responsive service, without abandoning traditional values. Indeed, some measures, such as the introduction of automated information systems, which facilitate consistent application of rules across the country, can contribute positively to both productivity and fairness.

In the UK, the first report of the Committee on Standards in Public Life (1995) lists the seven principles which should govern conduct in public life as:

1. selflessness
2. integrity
3. objectivity
4. accountability

5. openness
6. honesty
7. leadership.

The report states that 'these principles apply to all aspects of public life. The Committee has set them out here for the benefit of all who serve the public in any way.' Citizens are concerned, in the general sense, that the standards they expect from those they receive service from are being observed. In addition, individuals and individual organisations are expected to be accountable for their actions.

Wall (1996) quotes a number of sources to illustrate that answerability is not enough, and goes on to state that there seem to be three main ideas underpinning the concept of accountability: first, advocacy of public values; second, protection of the public interest; and third, custody of public resources.

The Department of Health framework

The Department of Health in Ireland has, in recent years, addressed comprehensively issues of strategy, structures and accountability which provide a good context in which the development and delivery of public health services in Ireland can take place in the period ahead. The stated primary aim of the strategy (*Shaping a Healthier Future*, 1994) is to enhance the health and quality of life of the people of the state. It adopts the concepts of health gain and social gain as the means by which improvements in population health will be pursued. Equity, quality of service and accountability are the principles underpinning the strategy. The Health (Amendment) Act 1996, commonly known to many in the health services as the 'accountability legislation', is intended to strengthen the arrangements governing the financial accountability of Health Boards and to clarify the respective roles of the members of Health Boards and their Chief Executive Officers. In this way the key questions of accountability – 'to whom?', 'for what?' and 'in what manner?' – are addressed. The concepts of health gain and social gain clearly suggest that improvements are attainable, and it follows that the pursuit of improvements involves the taking of calculated risks.

These developments are of interest in the context of the issues discussed in this chapter. Under the new legislation, Health Boards are required to secure the most beneficial, effective and efficient use of resources and to co-ordinate their activities with other health boards, local authorities and public bodies and to give due consideration to the policies and objectives of Ministers and the Government. In practice, the reconciliation of strategic goals (which may of necessity be long-term) with political goals (which in practice tend to be short-term) may give rise to problems. It is significant that legislation recognises the need to accommodate potentially conflicting goals in this way. The Act provides that certain functions, known as 'reserved functions', will be carried out directly by the members of the Health Boards. Any function which is not provided for in law to be a reserved function will be performed by the Chief Executive Officer and the staff of the board, and will be known as an 'executive function'. The basis of the accountability relationships between the Chief Executive Officer and the Health Board, and between the Health Board and the Department of Health, will in future be the 'service plan'. This plan will be prepared by the Chief Executive Officer and the staff of the board, but must be adopted by the board. It is also a function of the board to supervise the implementation of its service plan, in order to ensure that the net expenditure does not exceed the amount determined by the Minister. Alterations to the service plan also require the specific approval of the board. The Act requires the Chief Executive Officer to implement the service plan of the Health Board and to ensure that the net expenditure and indebtedness of the board do not exceed the amounts determined by the Minister. This provision has the potential to create tension between the board and its Chief Executive.

An interesting feature of the Act is that if the net expenditure incurred by a health board is greater or less than the amount determined by the Minister, the Health Board shall charge such excess or credit the amount of such surplus in its income and expenditure account for the next year. The accounts of Health Boards are now audited by the Comptroller and Auditor General, who reports to the boards and the Minister. The Minister lays the accounts before the houses of the Oireachtas, where they are scrutinised by the Public Accounts Committee.

Service plans – enabling or controlling mechanism?
The service plan has the potential to be a powerful vehicle for achieving measurable health and social gain, but it will take time to realise that potential. There is a real danger that because the service

plan has its origins in accountability legislation it will be perceived as a controlling rather than an enabling mechanism.

In its present undeveloped state, the service plan is more a service agreement. In its developed state the plan will consist of three inextricably linked elements – the finance resource component, the human resource component and the service component. The challenge is to achieve the balance which will result in the service plan becoming the vehicle for achieving measurable health and social gain.

Viewed in relation to the issues of risk management and accountability, the health services strategy, new legislation, and management development initiatives taking place go a long way towards achieving the balance necessary between encouraging risk-taking and satisfying the accountability expected of the public sector.

Adding value and satisfying changing accountability requirements

Where there is an over-emphasis on the need to be accountable, the danger of incurring what Drucker regards as the greatest risk of all – rigidity – is increased. When an organisation or the management of an organisation is perceived as being rigid, demands that the organisation or its management be replaced may result. The replacement approach runs the risk that what was admirable, from a prudent accountability point of view, in the old arrangements may be overlooked in assembling the replacement arrangements. The absence of accountability mechanisms, discarded in the name of progress and modernisation, may expose the new management or the new organisation to unacceptably high risks. The damage caused when the risk is incurred can result in not only the credibility of the organisation and the management concerned, but also the credibility of other organisations and management in that sector, being devalued. The challenge is to add value, through innovation, increased efficiency and effectiveness, and to go on doing so while satisfying changing accountability requirements.

The future

In seeking a balance between risk-taking and accountability, the rate of social change being experienced makes the risks of committing present resources to future expectations very challenging. Drucker (1994) believes that what he calls 'the age of social transformation' is not yet over and that the challenge coming may be more serious and more daunting than the challenges posed by the social trans-formations that have already come about. The form of balance he sees as necessary to cope with the social transformation we face is radically different to what has passed for balance up to now. If Drucker's vision of the future proves to be accurate – and his record suggests he is more entitled than most to have his predictions taken seriously – then what constitutes balance will have moved to a much higher and more interesting plane.

Having begun by quoting something Drucker wrote in 1973, let me end with food for thought by quoting something he wrote in 1994.

Organisations must competently perform the one social function for the sake of which they exist – the school to teach, the hospital to cure the sick, and the business to produce goods, services or the capital to provide for the risks of the future. They can do so only if they single-mindedly concentrate on their specialised mission. But there is also society's need for these organisations to take social responsibility – to work on the problems and challenges of the community. Together these organisations *are* the community. The emergence of a strong, independent, capable social sector – neither public sector nor private sector – is thus a central need of the society of organisations. But by itself it is not enough – the organisation of both the public and the private sector must share in the work.

CHAPTER 9

Managed Care and Healthcare in Ireland

Maureen P. Lynott

Introduction

Firstly, what is the management of care? In its conceptual and practical application, it encompasses structures, arrangements and frameworks which support:

- economic use of resources
- quality and effectiveness of care
- assurance and promotion of best practice
- reciprocal agreements and arrangements between providers of care and financers of care
- macro and local planning of the supply and growth of services
- the involvement of users of care in maintaining their own health and using health services appropriately.

The relevance of 'managed care' in the Irish context and other contexts is quite straightforward and essential: that is, to maintain access to high-quality care at an affordable cost, either via Exchequer funding of public health services or via voluntary/private health insurance funding. The macro factors affecting most health systems internationally are the same as those in Ireland: ageing, increases in length of life, increases in patient expectations, major advances in treatments and technology. The challenge is to provide access to high-quality affordable healthcare to a gradually ageing population.

Solutions will vary according to models, culture, and philosophy. Health policy-makers and financers, whether in state systems or voluntary/private insurance systems, have moved in recent years from an arm's-length position to a key role in developing frameworks with providers of care for benefit structures and payment methods which maximise current resources, promote best practice and prudently plan the growth of services – that is, which 'manage care': the quality, cost, efficacy and supply. What is interesting is that in spite of the diversity of funding and delivery models internationally, there is a similarity of issues relevant to healthcare financing and delivery. These issues apply internationally and in Ireland: management and organisation, quality and effectiveness, cost and affordability, availability and access.

Background in Ireland

In Ireland in the mid and late 1980s, both public health services and voluntary insured health services experienced significant financial strain and cutbacks. The cost increase of services was far in excess of the Consumer Price Index, volume growth and price increases. There were significant differentials in use and charges/costs for services and episodes of admission to hospitals. The latter could be partially explained by differences in case mix, specialisation, capital costs and development for hospitals, and how depreciation was charged, and by the fact that some hospitals traditionally did not cost for certain items. However, an analysis of length of stay for major causes of admission also showed significant variances among hospitals – this applied even with adjustments for the mix of cases and case intensity/severity in different hospitals. At that time, there was a perceived crisis in the financing and delivery of the health services, an absence of relevant data or controls regarding efficiency and best practice etc., and an absence of medical consultants in management and clinical audit/review. At the same time, hospital and health service managers were dealing with quite valid hospital operational needs and pressures while attempting to provide a good standard of care, meeting demand for services, developing services, and meeting requirements both for more primary and preventive care and for more complex treatment and equipment. Some of the problems related to the absence of information about the appropriateness and/or cost-effectiveness of various procedures. Additionally, there were problems of poor co-ordination among providers and across sectors of healthcare; a lack of incentives for efficient service provision; a lack of adequate information about the cost, quality and outcome of services; inadequate management of capital resources; and insufficient or inappropriate management at institutional level.

141

When one looked at comparability between providers, it was clear that the financing systems were reimbursing inputs, not outputs; providing incentives that did not sufficiently support efficiency; and financing significant differences in use of resources, practices and utilisation. A central question to the economic management of resources is: what are the incentives provided by the financing system for hospitals, doctors, and users/patients? It was concluded at that point, by public and insurance financers of hospital care, that the financing methods employed did not provide suitable incentives and it was necessary to move from retrospective financing to increased 'prospective financing' – i.e. the out-turn of payment to hospitals or basis of out-turn is agreed in advance, whether by annual budget, episode or case, case mix, efficiency adjustments, effectiveness adjustments, or a combination of these. Thus, the providers of care and the financers of care have a more shared investment and responsibility for the standards and cost of care – the beginnings of 'managing care'.

Supply and use of healthcare services

The public too have a role in 'managing care', and need to be educated that healthcare is costly and why, and that more or costlier care does not necessarily mean better healthcare or, indeed, better health. Richard Hamer, Director of Inter Study in the USA, states that 'studies show that up to one third of health care doesn't benefit health' and that in the USA 30% of all medical care is spent on the elderly in the final 60 days of life, with a significant amount of that spent prolonging death for people who are dying. The USA also has low patient satisfaction while spending more of Gross Domestic Product (GDP) for healthcare than any other country. In the State of Oregon, the first state in the USA to set priorities for funding of treatment, the main reasons why people visit a doctor are common colds, viral throats, soft tissue pain and lower-back pain. As a result, Oregon decided not to include treatment for the common cold in its healthcare package; the plan pays for the diagnosis of the cold but not for follow-up treatment. Incentives are in place instead to have patients informed about self-care for common ailments, or to steer patients with common complaints to a nurse practitioner rather than to a GP or specialist.

To the extent that they are not direct 'payers', people may not know or be affected by how much healthcare they utilise or how much it directly costs (while they would be sensitive to increases in the cost of taxes for health services or the cost of health insurance premiums). RAND, the research organisation, compared a group of people with insurance cover of 100% with a similar group whose insurance had a large annual deductible, i.e. an out-of-pocket or excess payment by the insured patient before insurance reimbursement applies. The fully insured group spent 40% more on healthcare, with no objective improvement in the health of the average member.

To the extent that cost of care is paid for by insurers or by government, individuals are relatively insulated from the costs of healthcare decisions made by them or, more likely, by doctors on their behalf. Supply, i.e. quantity and range of health services, is crucial to utilisation and cost of health services, and the 'balancing' of supply in relation to medical need (demand) is fundamental to managing care. In the normative marketplace, market 'need' – the extent and range of consumer/user demand for a service, product or commodity – can generally be relatively defined and quantified. Healthcare, however, does not conform to the dynamics of the marketplace in that demand may be generated by the user, but equally or more so may be generated by a provider or supplier of healthcare services. Medical *need*, then, may be construed as the *demand* for healthcare services and supplies by medical practitioners on behalf of the consumer, or by the consumer/user's desire or requirement for healthcare services.

A true complexity of the healthcare economy is that medical need or demand is generated by a user/patient, but significantly by a supplier who orders tests and services, carries out visits and treatments, refers for additional healthcare services, etc. This is a fundamental distortion of the dynamics of a marketplace economy in that both the consumer and the supplier generate demand, which may not necessarily be need, and have different though strong interests in doing so – the consumer or patient for their well-being and healthcare needs, relief of pain or symptoms, meeting of cultural expectations regarding care, etc.; the provider or supplier in relation to providing professional quality care, but also (and this must be part of the understanding of healthcare economy) out of a financial interest in supplying healthcare. Therefore, the provision of supply of healthcare services is crucial and must be carefully and objectively balanced to true medical need: what range of healthcare services should be provided; what are the proportions for acute hospital care, community and preventive care and self-care; what inventory of services is needed for a population; how much service might a population need?

Supply of healthcare must be economically planned such that sufficient is available but not an oversupply or an inappropriate mix of supply, which invariably results in overuse and overcost, or inadequate provision to meet medical need. Supply should reflect the health characteristics of the population being served, demographic characteristics such as age and gender, epidemiological characteristics, and assessment of an inventory of healthcare services which will most substantively address the strategic objectives for health services in a national or regional area. Are these objectives, for example, a reduction in hospitalisation, a reduction in mortality, an improvement in child health, development of community care, health gain? This aspect is a key responsibility of healthcare policy-makers in consultation with providers of care, financers, and those involved in the wider political process. Studies in the USA have demonstrated that a patient was more likely to receive appropriate and 'successful' care in a teaching hospital. Other studies suggest that where there are more surgeons per square mile, more surgery is performed – in other words, that at a certain point demand follows supply, not always need. Grenelle Bauer-Scott (1992) explores the issue of financing healthcare, whether via public finance or private insurance, and its impact on supply and demand. Exchequer health funding and health insurance tends to increase the demand for care, and can make this demand almost infinite:

> such financing reduces or eliminates for the patient the cost associated with the benefit, a situation which can be expected to increase demand. The more complete the coverage, both in terms of conditions covered and degree of coverage, the more the system can be expected to increase demand. While such financing tends to increase demand, medical science and advance in technology in medical equipment and pharmaceuticals are constantly expanding the potential supply of health care. This situation suggests the possibility of a continuous upward spiral of demand and supply. In these circumstances, i.e. almost unlimited demand in a rapidly increasing potential supply, the system appears to reflect an instance of market failure leading to oversupply... at the same time, it may also lead to under supply for those with inadequate coverage [or inadequate access].

What is managed care?

It is important to get behind some of the myths or stereotypes regarding 'managed care', particularly as it is perceived as operating in the USA.

Healthcare everywhere is delivered or managed in the context of national/regional culture, ethos and political structures. Very few models internationally are identical or highly similar. In Europe, in fact, 'management of care' has operated widely in the past decade, at least at a macro level, with varied forms of prospective financing, planning and regulation of supply, providers having a role in the cost of care via incentives and disincentives, setting of healthcare priorities, and increased use of relevant information on cost, outcome, and comparability. 'Managed care' is an expansion and development to include a continuum from macro through to micro/local care and through to direct patient care. Managed care means:

- co-ordinating integrated healthcare delivery for a patient
- managing for better quality, not just managing to control costs
- utilising relevant information to plan, deliver and modify services such as medical peer review and clinical audit, development of practice guidelines and protocols, outcome information, efficacy and efficiency analyses, patient satisfaction information
- providing incentives for primary care or outpatient care for both those who deliver and those who use care
- providing incentives for group arrangements for medical practices and hospitals, with joint planning and sharing of expertise and resources.

The USA is an insurance-based system for access to care. It is not a full entitlement system such as the United Kingdom, a mixed alternative system such as Ireland, or a compulsory insurance system such as Germany and other European countries. Insurance in the USA is either publicly financed for those who are very poor or elderly, or privately financed through non-profit and profit-making insurance, procured through traditional employer-paid benefits or purchased by individuals. Thirteen per cent of the American population – some 34 million people – are non-insured and are 'medically indigent'. Their lack of access to care and the resultant public health 'costs/ consequences', along with the real cost of obtaining emergency access to care, force unanticipated costs which are invariably shifted to

145

insurers. Further, in the USA, while the Federal Government regulates the Medicare and Medicaid systems for the elderly and the poor, each of the individual states then devises its own regulatory system for the operation of private and voluntary insurance. The system is highly fragmented and varies significantly between states in philosophy, objectives, degree of regulation, comprehensiveness, etc.

In the USA, a high profile has been given by Government and the public to universal access to medical care, and a reduction in the cost of care to both the individual and the employer, while maintaining a high level of quality and resources for care and avoiding what is perceived as 'socialised medicine' along the UK and Canadian lines. In the USA under typical pre-paid managed care plans, an individual or employer (or both) pay the plan a fixed amount to provide healthcare for a certain set of services/benefits over the course of a year. The doctors working for the plan are paid a predetermined fee in various ways: according to the number of patients they care for (capitated), or salary, or a fixed discounted fee for service. The doctor may work full- or part-time for the plan, or may be a designated participating doctor, in private practice, for one or several plans. Hospitals participating with a sole managed care plan are rare, unless owned by the plan (such as Kaiser-Permanente on the west coast, which is one of the oldest and most respected managed care organisations in the USA). More likely is a group or alliance of hospitals affiliated to a managed care plan or plans in a structured relationship regarding service levels, utilisation review, cost, etc., and reimbursed on some form of prospective basis.

In the USA, managed care also means managed competition between providers of care. Managed care plans compete for contracts to care for groups and individual patients, publicly and privately insured. Health maintenance organisations (HMOs) are a form of managed care and are likely to have systematic review of the activities and costs of their participating doctors and hospitals. Some studies have found cost to be substantially lower in HMOs than in open choice plans in a variety of settings, with high patient satisfaction.

The experience in America varies significantly: for example, on the east coast, managed care remains relatively suspect in terms of private/voluntary insurance where the individual medical practitioner has been the traditional method of delivery. However, in the western parts of the USA, and the west coast in particular, managed care in some form is very common and well thought of. Models for managed care in the US vary widely: some work well in regard to care and cost, some do not. There is not a uniform definition or model for managed care in the USA, or anywhere else for that matter.

Managed care: building blocks and process

'Managed care' may be perceived as restricted choice, rationed treatments and resources, lack of access to certain specialists, and price being placed ahead of quality. However, managed care does not imply a clinic or centre; neither does it necessarily mean reduced quality, administrative interference, approvals for hospital admissions and treatments, reduced price equalling reduced quality, poor choice, etc. It can take various forms.

Managing care is having in place structures, arrangements and frameworks which support the six elements listed at the beginning of this chapter. *The key element is joint reciprocal arrangements between providers and payers.*

The process for developing 'managed care' methods and models must include the key constituents and influencers: policy-makers, financers, providers, the public and those involved in the political process. Managed care cannot be imposed. It must be clearly thought out and addressed, and must include:

- clarity of objectives
- meaningful information
- a strategic focus
- incremental planning
- time – for consultation, dialogue, piloting, development
- monitoring and feedback.

First, *the objectives should be clear and widely agreed*: to provide appropriate high-quality services; to assure the financial solvency of the health services; to assure fair and sufficient payment to providers; to establish a clinically coherent system; to provide a useful management tool; and to develop a solution that is appropriate and fits with the Irish context and culture.

For users of care, the system should enable access to and adequacy of necessary care, as well as facilitating wellness, prevention and self-care of one's health. For providers of care, the structure should facilitate equity in payment, payment for resources and

147

renewal, administrative feasibility, reinforcement for good organisation and efficiency of care, reinforcement for positive outcomes, reward for case intensity. For financers of care, the system should facilitate comprehensiveness of care, effective outcomes, cost containment and relative predictability, and comparability of cost and inputs.

There is a very fundamental question of costs and benefits, not one where there is some administrative 'quick fix'. Real management of care and its resources means coming to terms with the notion that not all care is needed or sufficiently efficient/effective or of sufficient priority in the specific context. This means that choices must be made – informed decisions based on clarity of objectives, policy and outcomes.

Information is the foundation. At a micro and local level, timely information that provides a basis for clinicians and management to assess resource inputs, outputs and outcomes in terms of agreed objectives is essential: for example, improved patient health, reduced mortality, increased or decreased utilisation and throughput of services. Relevant information is essential to meaningful dialogue, the process of decision-making and change, and the process of 'managing care'. Information required includes comparative measurement and reports of outcomes such as length of stay, morbidity, improvements in various health indicators, cost ratios, case intensity, efficacy of alternative methods of treatment, technology and drugs, supply/medical need analysis. The last item is significant: there can be no 'management of care' without planning and balancing real healthcare demand/need with the supply of services, both in range and in quantity. This is where the political process and public opinion are crucial at a macro level and in influencing the micro level of healthcare delivery. One of the essential themes running through the Department of Health document *Shaping a Healthier Future* is that decisions on priorities and on the allocation of resources should be made in a more open and objective way, and should draw, in particular, on detailed information and analysis of health needs, costs and outcomes. This is vital, but the priority-setting process can never be made entirely objective; decisions will still need to be made in relation to the relative value of these benefits, i.e. choices must be made by those in positions of public responsibility both politically and for healthcare. Thus dialogue, feedback and information are integral to what must by its nature involve political as well as healthcare/clinical decisions.

Table 9.1. Policy approaches to changing a healthcare system

Demand side	Supply side
Indirect mechanisms	*Indirect mechanisms*
Cost sharing	Payment systems
Payment incentives in primary care	Provider markets
	Evidence-based purchasing
Demand management	*Changing service delivery*
Appropriateness and utilisation review	Development of management capacity
	Performance management techniques
Disease management	Cost reduction/efficiency programmes
Substitution policies: primary, community, home and social care strategies	Treatment protocols
	Quality improvement techniques
	Planning approaches
	Hospital closure
	Reconfiguration programmes

Source: Hensher & Werneke (1995).

Table 9.1 outlines macro policy approaches for restructuring healthcare financing and provision. Macro policy is the framework within which managing care occurs, and the management of care cannot take place effectively unless the macro policy framework of the relevant health care system supports this.

What can be done next in Ireland to move the process further towards managed care?

In 1994 the Department of Health published the first strategic plan for Irish health services (*Shaping a Healthier Future*). The strategy was based on three principles: equity, quality of service and accountability. It details strategic objectives for health gain, health promotion and prevention, treatment and care, and broadening the priority-setting process in allocation of healthcare resources.

The document is a substantive framework for the ongoing planning and delivery of care in Ireland. As a framework it has facilitated Government priorities in regard to action and resources and has contributed to reform initiatives in Irish healthcare which seek to address essential areas of development in order that the strategic principles which are established are incrementally achieved. Assessment of clinical efficacy is being developed; clinical costing and activity systems are being explored; regionalised planning is becoming more widely practised; an Office of Health Management has been established to address the need for increased depth and strength at all levels in the Irish health services; value-for-money auditing is occurring.

Ten issues to address in Ireland in order for managed care to 'work'

1. Comprehensive primary care integrated with higher levels of care, including relevant and appropriate prevention and screening programmes.

2. Defined specialist arrangements and organisation of clinical work, within and outside of hospitals.

3. Inter-hospital service planning and co-ordination, with financing and service agreements which emphasise primary care, out-patient services and day care around a core of acute care services.

4. Clinical protocols and clinical review along with increased integration of clinical services and budgets.

5. Strengthening management at all levels in the health services, and including clinicians in management as planners and decision-makers with both authority and responsibility.

6. Increased decentralisation of management and service delivery with clear standards for quality, cost and service levels.

7. Managing demand and utilisation, and planning the supply of services, i.e. setting priorities at national and regional level.

8. Protocols for planning and introduction of new technology and drugs based on sound epidemiological and research studies.

9. Relevant, timely user and policy information, particularly evidence-based outcome information.

10. Consumer education and information about prevention, wellness and self-care, and assessment of user satisfaction.

All health systems are strongly influenced by the underlying norms and values of their broader society. Within Ireland, the process of 'managing care' is under way. While there is no doubt as to the standard of clinical care in Ireland, we are all aware of 'spottiness' across the continuum of care – in management, in the lack of integration of care, the absence of rigorous planning and assessment, and deficits in co-ordination. For affordable, accessible, quality healthcare to evolve in Ireland to meet emerging demands and possibilities, the ten issues above must be addressed (and several are receiving serious attention currently) by health policy-makers, managers and providers in a focused and integrated way. Particular attention should be paid to the process of change, the underlying social values of equity in Ireland, the need for dialogue, and the importance – indeed urgency – of such change in regard to quality and availability of healthcare to the Irish people.

CHAPTER 10

Quality in the Irish Healthcare System

Austin L. Leahy

Introduction

Healthcare organisations throughout the world are focusing on quality of service. Substantial time, energy and resources are being devoted to improving quality at all levels. Healthcare providers, their administrative support, and companies which supply goods and services to providers are increasing their efforts to involve workers at all levels in making constant improvements to underpin quality.

In tracing the developments within the Irish healthcare system concerning quality, one must take cognisance of the special influences that the demographics and funding of health in Ireland exert. In the 1990s, quality improvements have been sporadic and individually driven. The development of central policy has received a renewed impetus with the publication of the Department of Health's strategy document, *Shaping a Healthier Future*. The development of a quality-based culture within the health system will place many challenges before management.

What is quality?

There are many definitions of quality. For any given individual, the only important definition is their personal interpretation of the quality of goods or services. While it is useful to dwell on definitions of quality, it is more important to recognise that there are many different views of quality. Inevitably, quality is a dialogue which must take place between the producers and users of a service. Within healthcare, therefore, three views of quality must be taken into account:

1. *the professional's view*, e.g. the view of the health provider (doctor, nurse, etc.)
2. *the manager's view*, which includes all the administrative support structure to the healthcare providers (hospital administration, Department of Health, politicians, etc.)
3. *the customer's view*, or that of patients and their relatives.

Quality has been defined as 'fitness for purpose' and 'conformance to requirements'. Within healthcare, a useful definition of quality is 'doing the right thing right consistently to ensure the best possible clinical outcome for patients, satisfaction for all customers, retention of talented staff and a good financial performance'.

Robert Maxwell of the King's Fund has defined quality in healthcare under six headings, as follows.

1. *Effectiveness* or technical competence: the successful outcome of treatment. Often this is the area which a professional emphasises.
2. *Social acceptability*: a particular concern to patients and their relatives.
3. *Efficiency*, or the need to deliver a service for the lowest unit cost.
4. *Availability*, or accessibility, which is an important societal measure of the quality of healthcare.
5. *Relevance*, indicating that services being offered are tailored to the needs of both the individual and society.
6. *Equity*, indicating the equality of access to services (Maxwell, 1997).

Clearly, any given service in the health system can be evaluated using these parameters. Inevitably, there are trade-offs between them. Effectiveness may require provision of high-tech equipment in a tightly regimented environment. This can limit social acceptability, with the patient and relatives being frightened by the technology and restricted in their role by the environment.

For any given service, in assessing quality, it is important that an attempt be made to maximise all the parameters of quality. The challenge to management is to recognise the many dimensions of quality and to engage in a dialogue between the professional, the patient and the manager.

Why become involved in quality?

There are many compelling reasons why individuals, managers and organisations are striving to increase quality in healthcare provision. The most frequently quoted include the following.

1. *Improvement in healthcare.* Best health outcomes are likely to be achieved by improving the quality of our services.
2. *Ethical reasons.* Working in the healthcare industry inevitably carries the responsibility of caring for people. Anything less than best quality performance in any given case is a disservice to patients.
3. *Financial allocation.* The elimination of waste saves money. With the world-wide attempts to control expenditure on health, the responsibility for spending money on doing the right things right has increased. Managers must recognise the responsibility to keep some of this aspect, while not losing sight of the other reasons.
4. *Accountability.* It is no longer sufficient for healthcare organisations to affirm a commitment to quality. Society, and in particular healthcare providers, the Department of Health and patients or patient organisations, demand built-in effective strategies for ensuring quality.
5. *Research and training.* There is an increasing need for quality assurance to be a part of training. The Royal College of Surgeons in Ireland, for example, refuses to recognise any training position which does not incorporate a commitment to audit and quality improvement.
6. *Retention of talented staff.* The best healthcare professionals are encouraged to work in organisations which are continually striving to improve. In contrast, failure to ensure quality is demotivating.
7. *Job descriptions.* Many contracts within the Irish health system now demand a commitment to quality initiatives by the employee.

The quality conundrum

It becomes important at this point to recognise the disparity between the simple tenets on which quality is based and the complexities involved in applying quality to a system such as the Irish healthcare system. In its simple form, quality is good for patient care, reduces waste and is therefore more economical, and is readily embraced by healthcare workers. Were it that simple, there would be little challenge for management in the introduction of quality measures.

Unfortunately, the complexities of health and of healthcare organisations impose a number of disciplines on the development of quality initiatives. Management must recognise that resistance to quality is understandable. It is only by recognising the validity of individual and organisational resistance to quality that managers can formulate strategies for quality development in Ireland.

Resistance to quality

Much research has been devoted to understanding the individual's resistance to quality. There is a genuine feeling within the health system that 'we are different'. The complexity of the environment inevitably hampers the translation of quality initiatives from other sectors into health. A further manifestation of this is that outcomes can be very difficult to measure. This contrasts with industry, which can easily define the limits of acceptability. In healthcare, individual variation, expectation and the variability of disease processes must be factored into any measurement of outcome.

Healthcare providers work within a stressful environment, where well-developed coping mechanisms are required. This manifests in many ways, including the professional camaraderie that develops within teams and the support which co-workers extend when adverse events occur. The development of audit systems and quality assurance may be viewed as a threat to coping mechanisms.

On an organisational level, hospitals are professional bureaucracies within which each discipline is largely self-contained. The lack of dialogue between disciplines is a barrier to the development of quality, as it hampers the consideration of entire processes. At its simplest, this is seen in the reluctance of nursing staff to become involved in assessment of medical staff, and indeed the unwillingness of medical staff to seek the co-operation of nurses for this purpose. Managers must recognise that the culture of professional bureaucracy needs to be altered to ameliorate resistance to quality improvement.

Ireland now has one of the highest levels of medical litigation in the world. Frequently this is cited as a reason to suppress information on adverse events. For many who fail to understand it, risk management may be seen as more of a threat to the healthcare provider than a useful tool.

Financial considerations also affect our willingness to embark on quality initiatives. This manifests in many ways. A healthcare provider may fear a loss of personal income due to the exposure of inadequacies. At management level, quality may indicate areas where financial expenditure is required. This in turn may lead to political resistance.

Finally, at the most fundamental level within health, fear and blame are prevalent. Often quality assurance can be seen as an attempt to fix the blame, rather than to fix the process.

Overcoming resistance

The introduction of quality initiatives is inevitably an exercise in the management of change. This involves managers in unfreezing current processes, initiating change and freezing improved behaviour. To unfreeze current processes, it is essential for managers to take account of the resistance to change.

In designing a strategy which will address individual and organisational resistances, managers must strive to change the culture of hospitals into one which accepts the need to improve processes in a non-threatening environment. This can be assisted by the development of multidisciplinary teams.

In Ireland, it is important that quality initiatives be promoted nationally, not only on an organisational level but also between organisations. National accreditation should be available, initially on a voluntary basis, for quality schemes. Largely this can be performed within existing resources, utilising those who are already involved in audit initiatives and quality exercises. Ultimately, by changes in the healthcare environment, all workers can be increasingly committed to quality. This should be the major focus of management involvement.

In Ireland, at present, the way forward lies in two strategies:

1. development of comparative audit or quality assurance
2. initiation of continuous quality improvement, by identifying processes which require multidisciplinary scrutiny.

Clinical audit and quality assurance

A great deal of overlap exists between the terms 'clinical audit' and 'quality assurance'. Both may be described as a systematic and critical analysis of medical care, with the aim of improving patient outcome. They could include an analysis of procedures used in diagnosis and treatment, as well as the use of resources and resulting outcome.

Audit should involve a consistent assessment of the quality of

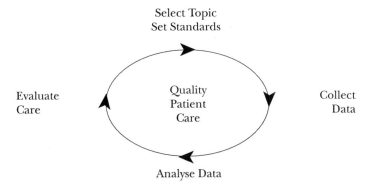

Fig. 10.1. The audit cycle

care delivered, comparing it with agreed standards. In essence, this is when audit and quality assurance become indistinguishable. This relationship is demonstrated in the audit cycle (Fig. 10.1). At the outset, acceptable standards of care are agreed. The audit process involves measuring the quality of care delivered and comparing it with agreed standards. If a deficiency is perceived, then systems must be put in place to reinforce the agreed standards, or else adapt them. This form of agreed standard has been referred to as 'benchmarking'. It allows the development of comparative data and the assurance of quality in relation to service delivery. For the purpose of this chapter, the term 'audit' rather than the term 'quality assurance' is used, as this is the more accepted term in Irish practice at present.

Realms of audit

There are numerous ways in which clinical audit can be classified. Donabedian has divided audit into areas of process, structure and outcome. Although this division is somewhat artificial, it points to the need for managers to consider more than just outcome. 'Process' refers to the systems through which patient care is carried out. 'Structure' refers to the available resources to deal with patient care. 'Outcome' refers to the results of treatment.

Medical audit has also been classified into four main types, as follows.

1. *Internal retrospective audit* is the simplest method of auditing medical care. It is internal to a speciality or a hospital, using past patient records to assess a particular condition or procedure.

2. *External retrospective audit* is when an outside group co-operates to implement audit. An example of this is a national mortality study, which allows all deaths to be evaluated by independent groups.
3. *Concurrent active audit* is a review of the care being given at present to patients, which is conducted in relation to established procedures or protocols. Utilisation review, which is practised in the USA, is a common form of this. It allows the management of patients to be compared with the care specified in clinical plans.
4. *Criterion-based audit* allows agreed explicit measured criteria of good practice to be selected.

Audit may be international; for example, the World Health Organisation collects data on infant mortality rates and uses them as an index of the well-being of health systems. International audit can measure only very definite end-points.

National or regional audit involves the application of audit programmes in a geographical area, allowing comparison between different centres. An example of this is provided by the Royal College of Surgeons in Ireland (RCSI) Surgical Audit Programme, where compatible audit was implemented in various units in three hospitals. Thus, units in different hospitals were compared.

Reports of the RCSI Audit Programme have been published, and clearly demonstrate a number of lessons for management. First, the confidentiality of the patient–doctor relationship must be respected. This can easily be achieved by an agreement that only aggregated data will be used by management. This is very much as outlined in the Gleeson Review of the Consultant Contract.

Second, management needs to recognise that audit should be adequately resourced. As well as supplying administrative personnel and information technology to support the audit, management has an ongoing responsibility to support the conclusions arising from audit meetings. In particular, where changes are indicated in the pursuit of quality, management must seek to achieve these changes.

Audit is inevitably a clinically driven initiative, and managers should cultivate those staff who are committed to audit. It is only by creating these champions within our hospitals and promoting individual effort that we can spread audit to other units.

Comparative audit systems

A number of audit projects are being organised on a regional basis in Ireland. These allow the comparison of data between hospitals, between units within hospitals, and between the areas of the Irish health service.

In considering how this may develop in Ireland, models from other systems can be studied. One such example is the Maryland Quality Indicator Project, which involves over 800 hospitals in the USA. Agreed benchmarks are implemented in an audit programme which assesses 16 indicators of the quality of the service. These include a number of indicators of outcome, including hospital-acquired infections, surgical wound infections, maternal mortality, neonatal mortality, and perioperative mortality. The Caesarean section rate, unplanned re-admission rate and unplanned admission rate following ambulatory procedures are assessed. Unplanned returns to a special care unit, unplanned returns to the operating room, and unplanned returns to the accident and emergency department within 72 hours of being seen are assessed. Also assessed are the requirement for patients to be treated in the emergency department for more than six hours, cases where discrepancies exist between initial and final diagnosis, and cases where X-ray reports require an adjustment in inpatient management. Patients who leave the emergency department prior to the completion of treatment are recorded, as well as the cancellation of ambulatory procedures on the day of the procedure. Data are analysed centrally. Where units fail to meet agreed standards, they receive assistance from units with better figures. This allows for a system of accreditation, which serves as an assurance of quality to the public.

Defining continuous quality improvement

If quality assurance involves protecting against unacceptable variances from defined standards, then continuous quality improvement involves immersing a healthcare organisation in a quality culture such that every area of the organisation is subjected to quality improvement. Thus, quality improvement involves a conscious, systematic and comprehensive strategy within an organisation aimed at raising the standards of care through improved work processes. Furthermore, reducing variation in performance and defining the processes more consistently results in improved patient care.

Figure 10.2 illustrates the Gaussian distribution of care which can relate to hospital stay, incidence of wound infection or, indeed, any other index of patient treatment. Quality assurance involves defining a benchmark and detecting processes that lie outside acceptable standards (Fig. 10.2a). Therefore quality assurance detects the exception or mistake. In contrast, by reducing unnecessary variation or unpredictability in the processes, and by continually attempting to improve standards, continuous quality improvement involves moving the bell-shaped curve to the left (Fig. 10.2b). This inevitably improves quality not only for those whose treatment lies outside accepted minimum standards, but for all patients involved in any particular treatment. Continuous quality improvement therefore has a much wider and more systemic impact on quality of care, but will equally prove to be a much greater challenge for management.

In the healthcare environment in Ireland, quality assurance programmes and audit systems are much better established than any attempt at continuous quality improvement. This has come about for a number of reasons. Most quality programmes are promoted by single disciplines, as it is easier for a group of surgeons or nurses to concentrate on variances in outcome. If processes are to be examined, a much more multidisciplinary approach is usually required. Frequently this is precluded by limitations in resources, and managers should

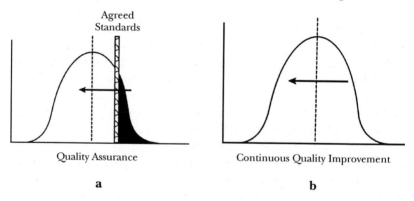

Fig. 10.2. (a) Audit or quality assurance detects the exceptions that fail to reach the agreed standards – by recognising their occurrence, quality can be improved; (b) continuous quality improvement examines processes for all, thereby moving the whole curve towards improved quality

consider a reallocation of existing resources to quality initiatives. It is also obstructed by a culture which builds barriers between professionals. Managers must develop strategies which overcome these barriers.

In the end it is the culture within our hospitals that determines how readily continuous quality improvement can be introduced. Ireland is not alone in recognising these difficulties and, in fact, it may take a generation for true continuous quality improvement to be introduced in healthcare.

Planning a continuous quality improvement strategy

A number of elements need to be implemented if management is to promote a quality improvement strategy.

First, there must be a commitment from the top. The leaders of organisations need to empower all departments and workers throughout the healthcare organisation so that it can be quality-driven. This requires not only an expressed commitment by management, but also the provision of adequate resources and channels for each voice to be heard equally.

Employees should be organised in quality improvement teams which work to tackle problems and analyse processes, thereby instituting new and better ways of working. As well as providing staff development in training, management must provide time to allow quality teams to meet.

Before processes can be examined, there must be a clear idea of customer priorities. Within the healthcare system a number of studies have been undertaken and a certain amount written about patients' views of quality. However, these studies frequently fail to obey the requirements of good market research. For example, if healthcare workers identified with the organisation are used to collect information, an incomplete picture of patients' requirements may result.

Management must emphasise the provision of good communications between workers, and indeed between quality teams. This is perhaps the single most important step in breaking down barriers imposed by professional power.

With these factors in mind, quality and continuous improvement can become an integral part of the workings of a healthcare organisation. The vital steps in the implementation of continuous quality improvement include the following.

1. Define patient expectations and translate these into priorities.
2. Examine processes and systems aimed at meeting the expectations of customers. Ideal processes are ones that meet the expectations of customers, enable staff to be effective, reduce stress in the organisation, are cost-effective and are clearly defined.
3. Managers must implement mechanisms within the organisation to allow effective quality improvement strategies to be implemented, leading to continuous improvement in standards while reducing lack of consistency.
4. Managers must strive to make the culture within the organisation supportive of continuous quality improvement. Ultimately there must be a move towards a 'seamless' organisation. This requires confidence-building measures, as it can threaten existing structures.

Continuous quality improvement in healthcare in Ireland

A number of organisations have expressed a commitment to continuous quality improvement and, indeed, have implemented programmes. Overall, however, the commitment is rather disappointing. Irish healthcare organisations are frequently top-heavy, professional bureaucracies. In this regard, senior members in each profession, including management, are frequently cautious about relinquishing power and are particularly resistant to multidisciplinary approaches to processes of which they feel ownership. It is also possible that quality improvement strategies are not seen to be adequately resourced and that the responsibility for implementing these strategies has not been seized by organisations. A major part in the development of continuous quality improvement would need to be the introduction of mechanisms to recognise the individual and team contributions to performance. This would go hand in glove with the development of incentives for organisations to move towards a quality approach.

The Department of Health needs to ensure quality, so that a quality assurance programme is both economical and reassuring. However, if the overall quality of the health system is to be improved and patient requirements addressed, continuous quality improvement must be instituted.

Strategy for Ireland

Central to the implementation of continuous quality improvement is the recognition that quality can only be improved by changing the culture of hospitals to allow multidisciplinary approaches. Management should achieve this through establishing regular meetings of 'quality circles' of professionals who all have a stake in the area being addressed. The area must be examined by concentrating on process improvement, identifying initially the less contentious processes. Multifactorial outcomes related to these processes must be identified. To put it simply, quality improvement should never become a witch-hunt. Problems must never be attached to personalities. Rather, it is important for management to find processes that can be improved.

Ultimately, managers need to change the culture of organisations. To unfreeze the current situation, which in many cases does not support process analysis, there must be a sensitivity to the resistances that exist.

While it is necessary for each hospital or group of healthworkers to define the processes that require improvement within their own area, it is worth while to give examples of areas that readily support this form of approach. It is hoped that management might find these processes to be less contentious areas, where a multidisciplinary team will not be seen as intrusive. Furthermore, these areas support the concept of multifactorial outcomes.

Communications within a hospital and between a hospital and its stakeholders (such as GPs) are an area that readily supports quality improvement. Within hospitals, there are already individuals and structures involved in communications. It should not be difficult for managers to create quality awareness by forming a team of some of these individuals.

The view from industry suggests that most unhappy customers do not offer complaints. Therefore their opinions on the quality of service must be sought, and this is a very useful area for teams to become involved in.

Discharge violations and admission violations are generally indicative of systemic problems, and should be of concern to management. Regular analysis of these problems can not only improve the quality of care to the customer, but also improve the working environment by defusing controversies.

Within certain departments, it may be possible to examine

quality. Two examples are the accident and emergency department and the records department. Within the accident and emergency department, for example, the throughput of patients can always be improved and therefore should be subject to continual examination, with processes being analysed and recorded. The records department in most hospitals can benefit from a similar continuous evaluation.

The whole concept of involving patients in their own treatments is central to the continuous quality improvement philosophy within hospitals. Patients should be provided with adequate information about their diseases, and they should be encouraged to seek more information and become fully involved in their own treatments. With the increasing shortage of nurses in the Western world, this will become not only a matter of benefit to the patients but also, perhaps, a matter of necessity.

A number of clinical protocols where multidisciplinary teams are involved would benefit from a continuous quality improvement approach. Examples include the management of bedsores, pain and specific conditions, such as rheumatoid arthritis.

While the above list is offered as an example of areas which support a quality approach, there are many more. Perhaps the best way for managers to begin introducing this philosophy into a part of the health system is to start with whatever processes are currently under their control, or they are currently engaged with.

Conclusion

Establishing a quality culture within the Irish health system will require continuing debate and compromise between the various stakeholders. Within that movement, management must recognise that individuals have a number of misgivings about the development of the quality approach and, consequently, these resistances should be addressed in framing developments. Institutions may also resist the implementation of a quality approach, specifically with regard to professions relinquishing power to more multidisciplinary groups. Management must stress that the movement towards a quality environment will be far more likely to improve the quality of the workplace for the employees and to reduce stress than the continuance of the current system.

Within Ireland, a reasonable strategy for managers to overcome resistance and move the quality agenda forward would include optimising the clinical audit programmes currently in existence and integrating them with other quality assurance systems in the healthcare system. Quality assurance departments would be an aid to successful implementation of these systems and would help to ensure that resources are being expended in the most effective and efficient way. It should be possible for management to provide an added impetus for quality assurance programmes by linking resource allocation to their successful implementation.

With regard to the establishment of continuous quality improvement, the establishment of multidisciplinary teams to examine processes is already under way in many of our hospitals. Management must formalise this, making quality improvement part of the framework of the health system.

PART FIVE

Managing in a Multi-Agency Environment

The Role of the Public Voluntary Hospital Sector in Shaping the Institutional Context of Health Policy in Ireland

PATRICIA BROWN

Introduction

This chapter examines the relationship between the public voluntary hospitals and state health policy. The transition from a residual charity-based to a state-funded health system was a gradual and slow process. It was a complex and challenging one in the Irish context due to a range of factors, including the reliance of the state on public voluntary hospitals whose tradition, ethos and legal character were essentially pre-statist. The institutionalisation of state hospital policy in the Irish context involved the gradual renegotiation and redefinition of how the 'public interest' and 'public accountability' would best be served.

An analysis of the Reports of the Hospital Commission (1933–47) shows a strong commitment to the role of the state health authorities in promoting the right of the community (and in particular the poorer sections of the community) to hospital care. There is clear acknowledgement of the state authorities' responsibility for ensuring that hospitals were accountable, and responsive to community health needs. These early Reports provide evidence that there was a well-worked-out concept of the state's role in regard to healthcare at that time. Equally, the Commission articulated how in practice the state might deliver on public accountability in healthcare, albeit in a devolved system. However, the analysis also demonstrates the reality of the 'bottom-up' character of the institutionalisation process, and the nature of the responsibility that the state health authorities had (in the early years of the state) in making the transition from charity to state healthcare.

The analysis of the period 1930–60 demonstrates the relevance of this earlier phase in the development of national policy to an understanding of some of the unique strengths of the current system, and outstanding problems and challenges facing Irish health policy-makers today.

The institutional context refers to the regulatory/legislative context or the formal rules governing a policy area. It also refers to organisational context and to the characteristics of the organisational infrastructure of service delivery, such as the diversity of the organisational context, the autonomy of the organisations, their ethos and culture, and the organisations' power base. These features of the organisational context are particularly important in the case of a service such as acute hospital care, where timeliness, responsiveness and equitable access to care are paramount.

The health status of the population

Up to the 1930s, state responsibility for healthcare was largely confined to the provision of primary and custodial care for the poor and some public health functions. The failure to implement a prepaid health insurance scheme in Ireland in 1911 in effect meant that statutory health services were to remain (until the 1960s), from the point of view of eligibility, restricted and means-tested. In her analysis of the reasons why the proposal to extend insurance to Ireland was eventually rejected, Barrington (1987) identifies the opposing interests as follows:

> on summary it can be said that insurance-based medical benefits were not introduced to Ireland for a combination of reasons among which the most important were the ill-conceived nature of the proposed medical benefit as it affected Ireland, the opposition of the hierarchy to the Bill, the determined resistance of influential sections of the medical profession, the financial implications of a reorganised system of general practice for a Home Rule Government, the poor leadership and organisation of the IMA representatives and the lack of will and ability of the Liberal Government to force the benefits on Ireland against the wishes of its representatives. (p. 165)

The economic conditions at the time are also important in accounting for the reluctance of the state to extend eligibility and to develop health services. However, there was at the same time a growing awareness among Irish policy-makers of the need to develop the health services and to provide a wider right of access to healthcare.

The health status of the Irish population relative to that of other European countries, including the United Kingdom, was a cause for concern. Poor economic conditions, poverty and malnutrition no doubt contributed to the rising rates of infectious diseases in Ireland. In relation to tuberculosis, for example, Barrington (1987) notes that:

> The death rate from tuberculosis in 1940, 1.25 per 1,000 was almost exactly the same as it had been in 1933. From 1937 onwards, the death rate from the disease began to show an upward trend, isolating Ireland from most European countries where rates were falling rapidly. (p. 129)

Maternal mortality, particularly outside Dublin, was very high. Infant mortality was also high and rising in the 1930s. According to Barrington (1987):

> At 66 deaths per thousand in 1939, the rate was about the same as in 1930 and was 16 deaths higher than for England and Wales. Cities and towns continued to experience a much higher fatality than rural areas. The problem was particularly serious in Dublin County Borough from a severe epidemic of gastro-enteritis: the death rate among infants would rise to 79 per 1,000 births in 1944 before anyone kicked up a row about it. (p. 132)

It is important to note this backdrop of alarming public health problems, exacerbated by extremely poor social conditions (poverty, malnutrition and poor housing), and limited eligibility to healthcare, in order to understand the significance of the shift towards a stronger decisive role for the central state authorities in health funding and planning in Ireland in the 1930s and 1940s.

In this context also, one might point out the more important contribution of preventive, as opposed to direct, health services. Much energy and effort went into developing preventive public health in the early years of the state. This aspect of health policy is not, however, the subject of this review.

Institutional health services were tainted by their poor-law history. The combination of extremely poor social conditions and high rates of infectious disease meant that institutional care had as much a social control (containment of disease) role as it had a custodial/humanitarian one.

The public voluntary hospitals had a much better image. Their independence from the state and their strong links with the medical profession and the religious were important factors. They enjoyed strong community support and, because of the identification and commitment of the medical profession with them, they also provided the highest technical standard of care.

The differences between the standards of care provided in the state hospitals and the independent voluntary sector became more apparent as developments in medical science increased the capacity of medical intervention to treat infectious and other medical conditions effectively and safely. These developments, in Ireland as elsewhere, transformed the role of the hospital from that of caring for the poor and destitute to providing cure as well as care for all social groups. The demand for care widened as drug therapy and other technical developments reduced the risks and dangers attached to hospital care, thereby making hospital care attractive to the working and middle classes.

Voluntary hospitals continued to provide for the poor, but increasingly they also faced demand from paying patients. Their dependence on the income from paying patients increased as their technical capacity increased. The establishment of the Sweepstakes fund was an effort to address what had become a funding crisis for voluntary hospitals as they ran up deficits in an attempt to cope with rising demand and costs.

The role of the Hospitals Commission: establishing state jurisdiction

The Hospitals Commission was something of a watershed in the evolution of the Irish state's role in and responsibility for health services. It was charged with the task of surveying hospital facilities in each area, of reporting on applications from voluntary hospitals for grants from the Sweepstakes funds, and with the power to inspect any hospital and examine receipts and expenditures. Its contribution was to confront directly the question of the role and responsibility of the state for the planning of hospital services for the community. This inevitably also revealed a conflict between the emerging concept of the state as guarantor of the community's (or individual's social rights of) access to social services, and that of the voluntary tradition of access based on the ethos or the character of private voluntary institutions (based on duty and an appeal to community values). The two are not necessarily incompatible, but they are based on very different values and assumptions, as the analysis of the Commission's Reports shows.

Many of the voluntary hospitals were established by charter, but not all were. For those that were, their charter provided a general undertaking to serve the poor. It addressed the requirement of community access by defining the hospital as a charitable institution with a core responsibility to serve the poor. Boards of voluntary hospitals had responsibility to ensure that the hospital remained committed to its social responsibilities to the poor. These charters defined public responsibility in terms of the institution's ethos and its duty to the poor, rather than in terms of recipients' rights (understandably, given its pre-statist origins). Access also depended on the capacity and admission policy of individual hospitals. These were not sufficient bases on which to develop and underwrite access by the community to public hospital care. This became increasingly apparent after the foundation of the state in the late 1920s and early 1930s, as demand for hospital care grew, and the cost and complexity of care increased. Donations, bequests, etc. declined and voluntary hospitals became increasingly dependent for their income on fees from paying patients. The Fourth Report of The Hospitals Commission (1938) described the limits of the voluntary hospital system as a model of public provision:

> Under the voluntary hospital system there was no legal guarantee that any sick person, and more particularly any sick poor person, needing hospital treatment would be admitted to a voluntary hospital. There was, however, a guarantee of another nature which although without any legal sanction, was nevertheless fairly effective. It was that these hospitals depended to a very large extent for their existence on the measure of public support which they received by way of subscriptions and donations, legacies and bequests of various kinds... and this support was liable to be adversely affected, if these hospitals could not show that they were rendering in return a fairly complete service for that section of the community which could not of their own efforts provide it. (p. 8)

The Sweepstakes, set up by the voluntary hospitals to deal with their funding crisis, was an outstanding success in generating income. The income from charitable donations etc. decreased further as the public became aware of this success. A large central fund in turn reduced the need for voluntary hospitals to engage in local fund-raising, and weakened the strong community sanction that characterised the relationship between voluntary hospitals and their communities. In fact, prior to the establishment of the Sweepstakes the voluntary hospitals had become more reliant on income from paying patients: for instance, Barrington (1987, p. 8) makes the point that 'The income from paying patients in six voluntary hospitals in Dublin averaged £2,000 a year before the war; in the 1920s the income had risen to an average of £24,000'.

The success of the Sweepstakes can be attributed to the ingenuity of the organisers in imaginatively tapping into local networks of Irish emigrants overseas. There was considerable and understandable resentment at the haste with which the state took over the Sweepstakes, and at its failure to help the voluntary hospitals pay off their deficits at an earlier stage. As the voluntary hospitals saw it, the Sweepstakes had been established by them.

The hospitals were surviving on a very voluntary basis with little or no state intervention. It was the funds from the Sweepstakes, and not taxpayers' money, that developed the county hospital system. However, the Commission was bureaucratic in its approach to the distribution of funds, allowing the hospital managers little or no discretion.

Access to public care in voluntary hospitals in the 1930s

There was some weakening of public confidence (among the poorer sections of the community) in the voluntary hospital system in the late 1920s and the 1930s, as the voluntary hospitals were perceived to favour paying over non-paying patients. The question of the right of access of poor patients to beds in public voluntary hospitals, particularly in the cities, where there was no alternative hospital care, was raised by the Commission in its reports.

In its First Report (1933, p. 58), the Commission, in setting out in detail the conditions to be attached to grants to hospitals from the Hospitals Trust Fund, emphasised the overriding concern: 'to produce a co-ordination of all hospital services functioning primarily in the interests of the poor without placing undue restrictions on the elasticity associated with the normal functioning of voluntary Hospital units'.

The Commission saw the question of guaranteeing the poor access to hospital care as a core responsibility of the state, and as an issue of public accountability. The saliency of this issue, referred to in several of the Reports of the Commission, in practical terms arose due to overall bed shortages, a possible tendency by voluntary hospitals to unintentionally under-serve poor patients (because of declining income from voluntary sources since the 1920s), and a growing public perception that paying patients had priority access, and that poor patients were not getting the access that the state had paid for on their behalf. These were very serious issues.

From the Commission's observations, it would seem that the question of unequal access was more than a matter of public perception. In its First Report (1933, p. 59) the Commission noted, for instance, that cases had come to its notice where:

> ... Local Authorities, Dispensary Doctors and General Medical Practitioners have telephoned one city hospital after another in order to secure a bed for a particularly urgent case only to be told by each that no bed was available. A series of such fruitless long distance calls means an additional expense to the Local Authority, apart altogether from the effect of the delay on the patient's health.

In the same report (p. 59) the Commission notes, in relation to the refusal to admit patients, that 'There is a general opinion abroad that this excuse (that no beds were available) covers a tendency on the part of the hospitals to discriminate against poor patients'.

The institutional structure of provisions: dual standards of care?

The question of access by the poor clearly went deeper than the technical issue of overall bed numbers. More worryingly, from a policy point of view, it revealed the early signs of dual standards of care, in so far as meaningful access to care for paying and non-paying patients differed significantly. This problem was reinforced by the existing institutional structure of provision.

The situation in Cork city, discussed in the Second Report, is instructive. The proposal from the management of the Union Hospital (state hospital) for a grant to develop a 400-bed acute medical and surgical unit raised the question of the appropriate strategy for co-ordinating and developing general hospital services in Cork city. The Commission favoured the development of the Union Hospital, plus the amalgamation of all or some of the existing voluntary hospitals.

In its Report, the Commission showed that only approximately 40% of the existing bed accommodation in Cork voluntary and semi-voluntary hospitals was utilised by city patients.

The proposal to develop a municipal hospital was discussed with the relevant interests, including the existing voluntary hospitals. Eventually it was agreed that a new hospital be provided, but 'only on condition that the right of the existing hospitals to substantial benefits from the sweepstakes funds was not interfered with' (p. 30).

The price paid for the development of the state hospital sector was the voluntary hospitals' unaltered claim on funds. This type of trade-off is recorded many times in the Reports of the Commission, illustrating the substantial power and influence the voluntary hospitals wielded at the time. In the case of Cork, the Commission's Second Report, in its review of the bed provision of the existing voluntary hospitals, noted that 'these hospitals do not appear to cater for the type of patient for which the Union Hospital caters' (p. 30).

One of the arguments put forward by those opposing the development of a large municipal general hospital, cited by the Commission, was that different institutions were required to treat the different classes of patients. The argument was summarised by the Commission (and rejected by it) in its First Report (pp. 30–31):

> ... that the class of patient catered for by those hospitals would not avail of treatment in a central hospital and that, therefore, they (voluntary hospitals) should be maintained for middle class patients. The Commission is not convinced that a modern General hospital would not attract to it patients of all classes. The maintenance of separate middle-class hospitals, as distinct from middle-class accommodation in a general hospital, is opposed to the principles of all modern hospital development. If however, such hospitals can be made self-supporting, there can be no objection to their continuance for the hospitalisation of selected classes of the community ... but such continuance at the expense of the poor could not be recommended.

The preferred policy option: an institutionally integrated system of care for all

The state authorities, as the Commission's analysis showed, were singleminded in the determination with which they insisted on establishing a policy framework for hospital policy that provided an institutionally integrated system of care for all social groups. Although the Commission may be criticised for its lack of success in rationalising hospital services, what it did achieve was arguably a more important objective: establishing an integrated and publicly accountable system of care for all. It is noteworthy that this was achieved despite the institutional diversity, the powerful position and independence of voluntary hospitals and their determination to retain a significant measure of independence, and the state's dependence on voluntary hospitals for acute hospital care.

The poor-law legacy had attached a stigma to attending state hospitals, which were former workhouses. The middle classes and anyone who could afford to, up to the 1960s, avoided what were sometimes referred to as 'public assistance hospitals'.

The widening of eligibility, particularly the abolition of the 'public assistance class', was the most significant development in state hospital policy. This change facilitated the integration of the system. The negative image of the public system was therefore due both to history and to the restricted eligibility for public care which reinforced class selection by institution. The voluntary hospitals were subject to these pressures in their environment, and perceived therefore by the general population to be superior to publicly owned hospitals. This is an important qualification.

Measurement-based accountability

The Commission (in spite of the limitations of working within a system of restricted eligibility for public care) established an integrated planning framework by establishing clear guidelines for the first time for the payment of hospital trust funds and insisting on what might now be referred to as 'measurement-based' accountability. In a devolved system, the Commission recognised how important a role mandated information returns would play (see section (h) of conditions for receipt of grants, First Report, p. 58) in improving the state's capacity to address accountability and achieve important planning objectives.

The Commission used statistical information on bed provision to investigate problems of co-ordination and resource use. For instance, information on bed occupancy and availability discussed in the Third Report demonstrates clearly that serious problems of access to care in Dublin were due in large measure to the uncoordinated closure of wards by voluntary hospitals during the summer months. Similarly, the Commission drew on statistical information on length of stay to query the use of resources (Seventh Report, p. 3). In the Seventh Report (p. 5), the Commission also drew attention to 'wide divergence in the figures of the cost per occupied bed of the individual institutions'.

On this question of cost per bed, the Commission's analysis, interestingly, showed that 'the cost per occupied bed in the lay controlled general hospitals is much higher than in the case of general hospitals controlled by members of a religious community' (Sixth Report, p. 5).

While the Commission was very concerned with improving efficiency and with accountability for cost, it also highlighted failure to address needs, and in this regard it was critical of the local health authorities' failure to provide adequately for the hospital needs of tuberculosis patients. Barrington (1987, p. 130) demonstrates the important role the Commission played in identifying unmet need:

> The annual reports of the department of Local Government and Public Health in the early 1930s hid behind the official figures for the number of approved schemes, dispensaries and beds set aside for tuberculosis patients. The cosy picture was broken when the Hospital's Commission surveyed the beds actively in use: there were 3,164 beds officially approved for tuberculosis, but only 2,686 available. The Commission pointed out that the Danes, with a death rate from tuberculosis that was half the Irish rate, had 1,000 beds more than their actual number of deaths. There were few beds for non-pulmonary cases in the Free State. Tuberculosis dispensaries, although charged with the task of diagnosing the disease, did not have X-ray equipment. Most of the sanatoria could not treat the disease as they lacked modern surgical facilities and some buildings were most unsuitable.

A central Bed Bureau was proposed by the Commission as a mechanism to improve central control and co-ordination of hospital beds and thereby ensure that the system was accountable and responsive to need, and that it was perceived to be so by the public. However, the bureau was not established. None the less, the principles underlying the proposal were accepted, and the essential nature of information and measurement for the management and co-ordination of a national – particularly, a devolved and partly independent – hospital system was clearly demonstrated.

It is important not to overstate the degree of control achieved by the state over the voluntary hospital sector. Voluntary hospitals retained their independence, their diversity and a good measure of power and influence within the system (see *Report of the Commission on Health Funding*, 1989).

The move away from a capitation payment system for voluntary hospitals in the 1950s, and its replacement with global budgets, increased the operating autonomy of the hospitals and their managers. It also unintentionally reduced the role of mandated information. Widening eligibility for health, particularly hospital services in the 1960s, underlined once again the need for a tighter planning framework that would facilitate the rationalisation of publicly funded hospital services. The growing national prosperity of the 1960s and 1970s allowed hospital services to expand without careful scrutiny of efficiency or cost issues. In the longer term, a strong information-driven approach to the management and co-ordination of public hospital services did not in reality materialise until the late 1980s.

Conclusion

The foregoing analysis helps to clarify why the co-ordination and integration of hospital services has proved to be, and continues to be, a formidable challenge in the Irish context: some of the key issues already identified in the Hospital Commission Report are revisited in the Kennedy Reports (Dublin Hospital Initiative Group, 1990, 1991). The problem of a fragmented, poorly integrated service is once again highlighted. Although they define the concept of an integrated service in broader terms, the Kennedy Reports place a considerable emphasis on a structural capacity to undertake an overall needs assessment of the community and to use information to determine patterns of demand, utilisation and cost – this finds echoes in the work of the Hospital Commission. The Kennedy Reports and *Shaping a Healthier Future*, in contrast to the Hospital Commission's approach, favour the decentralising of decision-making and a devolution of management functions to area level. The emphasis according to the Health Strategy (1994, p. 30) should be on 'devolved responsibility' combined with 'increased accountability ... and independent monitoring and evaluation of the performance of executive agencies'.

One of the challenges for hospital planning authorities is to achieve a balance between central policy co-ordination (control) and institutional responsiveness and dynamism (autonomy) at hospital level. A degree of tension or friction is inevitable in a system that is managed with this balance in mind. Central (state) dominance or institutional dominance from below are equally undesirable.

The history of the development of a national framework for hospital services in Ireland shows that state jurisdiction was contested and resisted and that compromises were worked out as the need for balance between the different interests involved was pragmatically recognised. Inevitably there were times when dominance, either by the state authorities or by interests at the institutional level, became problematic. The over-zealous approach of the Commission to information returns led to some criticisms of bureaucratic dominance. On the other hand, dominance of the public voluntary sector of the provision of acute hospital care in the period prior to the establishment of the 1933 Commission, and the hospitals' resistance (understandable as it was) to state control of the Sweepstakes fund, unintentionally threatened the interests of the rural poor, whose needs could not be met effectively without upgrading the existing network of county hospitals.

A strong dynamic infrastructure is compatible with an equally strong approach to policy co-ordination. This is one of the main lessons that the development of Irish hospitals reveals. The focus of policy energy and effort has to be on the balance and on maintaining this balance. Developments in measurement and information systems can facilitate the co-ordination of policy while allowing greater operating autonomy to hospitals, their managers, professionals and staff.

Measurement and information are important tools in a policy context where policy co-ordination and service delivery are at times contested terrain. The extent to which measurement will usefully mediate conflict will depend on the legitimacy of measurement-based management within the system and the extent to which the different interests within the system accept and identify with some core values and objectives.

CHAPTER 12

Changing Relationships and the Voluntary and Statutory Sectors

Tim O'Sullivan

Introduction

The OECD (1996) highlighted the work in Ireland of area-based partnerships of statutory and non-statutory bodies which are combating poverty and social exclusion. It suggested that the partnership approach followed in Ireland could have considerable potential for other countries as well – for example, in facilitating active participation by citizens in the decisions that shape their lives.

The importance of *partnership* in the health sector, between statutory and voluntary agencies, is a central theme of this chapter. Discussion of the voluntary sector and of statutory–voluntary relationships in health and social care is necessary in a book on health management because of the importance of the voluntary sector in this country. That sector, the Health Strategy noted in 1994, 'plays an integral role in the provision of health and personal social services in Ireland which is perhaps unparalleled in any other country' (p. 33).

This chapter examines changing relationships between the voluntary and statutory sectors in Ireland in the period up to and beyond the launch of the Health Strategy. It sets out the increased importance of the voluntary sector in Ireland and elsewhere in recent years, and examines key issues in voluntary–statutory relationships. The discussion below operates on the premise that the voluntary sector, as well as the state, makes an important contribution to the common good. However, while the important role of the state is generally well understood in public management literature, less attention has been paid to the specific justification for and role of the voluntary sector. This chapter therefore focuses to some extent on the voluntary sector and sets out some philosophical arguments for that sector, notably those reflected in the principle of subsidiarity.

The chapter includes in its definition of voluntary organisations both the large institutional providers – for example, the public voluntary hospitals and large mental handicap agencies – and smaller organisations, but some characteristics mentioned below (for example, the large volunteer resource of voluntary organisations) relate more to smaller organisations. Some current developments, for example, the publication of *Supporting Voluntary Activity* (1997), the Green Paper on the voluntary and community sector, also relate more to smaller voluntary organisations, while others – such as the reorganisation of health care in the Eastern Health Board – relate more to the state's relationship with the larger institutional providers. However, some common issues apply to both sets of voluntary organisation, including the nature and structure of their relationships with statutory bodies.

Growing emphasis on the voluntary sector

If more attention is being paid to the voluntary sector today, this is partly because of the crisis of the Welfare State. The role of the voluntary sector tended to be neglected in health and social policy literature before the 1980s, at least in the English-speaking world. Before this period, developments and problems in State provision generated social policy's academic agenda. Confidence about the future of the Welfare State was summed up in the 1970s by Gunnar Myrdal, a well-known Swedish welfare economist, who is cited by Johnson (1987):

> I see the welfare state as more than an achieved solution. Dynamically it has become an almost immutable trend. Its further development can be slowed down for a time and occasionally even slightly reversed. But after such a stop it can be expected to continue its course. (p. 29)

The voluntary sector suffered from benign neglect; it was seen as very marginal, even if worthy in its own way. However, important developments in the 1970s and 1980s led to a Welfare State crisis and therefore to a new interest in non-statutory solutions. These developments are summarised as follows by Johnson (1987, p. 40).

1. *Economic problems* such as lower growth, higher unemployment and lower rates of investment.
2. A problem of government growth, leading to what is sometimes described as *government overload.*

3. *Fiscal problems* – in other words, governments overstretching their resources by attempting too much, budget deficits being one result of this phenomenon.
4. *Legitimation problems,* which are intimately linked to the other three areas: according to Johnson, 'if, because of economic, administrative and fiscal problems, the welfare state cannot deliver what it promises, or what people expect of it, then it begins to lose mass support; there is a loss of legitimacy'.

It is important to note that Johnson is not attacking the Welfare State. He is arguing that because of a variety of technical problems, the Welfare State ran into serious problems; but his analysis does not seek to reject the role of the state.

With the crisis of the Welfare State, there was a growing acceptance in the 1980s of what is called welfare pluralism or the mixed economy of welfare, that is to say, an emphasis on sources of welfare provision apart from the State: in particular, the private market, the family and the voluntary sector.

The crisis in, and re-examination of, the Welfare State was very marked in Britain, and developments in Britain are important because they were influential elsewhere in the English-speaking world. In the 1980s the Thatcher governments, which espoused a militant pro-market policy, rejected accepted models of the state in social provision and, more specifically, an unquestioned dominant role for the state. Under Mrs Thatcher, as Wilding (1992) notes:

> All managers were supposed to live with certain basic questions never far from their lips. What are your aims and objectives? How are you setting out to achieve them? What do your various activities cost? What are the outcomes of what you do? (p. 111)

An implication of asking these very fundamental questions was that if one found, as a manager in a statutory organisation, that the most efficient way to meet one's objectives was to contract-out some aspect of one's service to a voluntary or private body, there was no reason in principle why one couldn't do that.

Mrs Thatcher's philosophy can be seen as pro-market and anti-state rather than as pro-voluntary sector in any deep sense. Nevertheless, the Thatcher era in Britain did result in the attachment of greater priority to the provision of services by non-statutory sources, and the British experience influenced interest in voluntary provision in other countries.

In summary, then: after a period of neglect, international interest in the voluntary sector has been increasing in recent years. This increased interest has been influenced by the crisis of the Welfare State and by a perceived need to examine sources of welfare provision apart from the state and to develop alternatives or supplements to state provision.

The voluntary sector in Ireland

Ireland has shared in the international trends just mentioned in relation to the voluntary sector, i.e. a relative neglect in the past and an increased emphasis in recent years on its role. O'Connell and Rottmann (1992) highlight the size and importance of the Irish Welfare State and argue that there was a major expansion of the Irish Welfare State from the 1960s. They state that the expansion of social rights in Ireland – i.e. rights to welfare, equality and security, to which citizens are entitled unconditionally – constituted a 'silent revolution' in this country (p. 205).

The voluntary sector is also very large in Ireland, and could never have been seen as marginal here. Nevertheless, it has arguably not received the priority that its size and importance would have warranted. Butler (1981) pointed to the lack of adequate statistics on the Irish voluntary sector in arguing that lip-service rather than genuine priority was given to voluntary activity in Ireland. The Council for Social Welfare (1991) highlighted a number of issues relating to the voluntary sector which (it argued) were unresolved for decades – the lack of any coherent social policy framework for the voluntary sector, the lack of partnership between the statutory and voluntary sectors, a 'labyrinthine' funding system and the absence of a clear concept of the role of the voluntary sector. In 1989, the *Report of the Commission on Health Funding* – arguably the most comprehensive analysis of healthcare funding and management ever produced as an official report in Ireland – highlighted the 'immensely important' role of voluntary organisations, but devoted only a couple of pages out of almost 400 to the specific issue of the role of voluntary organisations in Ireland.

Nevertheless, the international crisis of the Welfare State has contributed to a re-examination in Ireland as well of the role of the voluntary sector. In 1994, the Health Strategy stated that for the first time, a specific statutory framework would be created between the health authorities and the voluntary agencies and that this framework would recognise the role and responsibilities of both sectors.

Clearly, any discussion of the voluntary sector in Ireland must allude to its great diversity. Jaffro (1996) points to the influence of religious and self-help organisations in the nineteenth and twentieth centuries and to a more recent 'new wave' of community-based organisations, sometimes supported by EU funding.

Faughnan's (1990) classification of voluntary bodies gives some indication of their diversity:

- mutual support and self-help organisations (e.g. small local organisations)
- local development associations
- resource- and service-providing organisations (large bodies, such as the public voluntary hospitals)
- representative and co-ordinating organisations (e.g. the Disability Federation of Ireland)
- campaigning bodies (e.g. ISPCC)
- funding organisations (e.g. Trócaire).

Some would argue that large service organisations (such as the public voluntary hospitals or large mental handicap agencies), which receive most of their funding from the State, should be described as non-statutory rather than 'voluntary' organisations. Certainly there are enormous differences between a small local meals-on-wheels organisation and a large public voluntary hospital. Nevertheless, many voluntary organisations also share certain characteristics such as independent ownership and administration and a common need to develop appropriate relationships or partnerships with the state. In this chapter, as noted above, all agencies which are not directly owned or run by the state are included under the voluntary category. A similar broad definition is followed by the Health Strategy. Distinctions will be made, however, between issues that apply to the larger organisations and those that apply to the smaller organisations. For example, a given Health Board may provide token funding to a particular small voluntary organisation and very substantial funding to one of the large voluntary agencies operating in its region.

Comparative data on the size of the voluntary sector in different

European countries are difficult to obtain. Important comparative reviews of welfare policy – such as those of O'Connell and Rottman (1992), Ó Cinnéide (1993) and Hantrais (1995) – concentrate on the role of the state or of the EU and devote limited attention to the voluntary sector.

The size of the voluntary sector in Ireland is nevertheless worthy of note. In relation to the larger institutional providers, close to one-half of acute hospital beds and two-thirds of mentally handicapped residential places are provided by non-statutory organisations. In relation to social service organisations, 900 voluntary agencies involved in just one service area, the care of the elderly, responded to a survey reported by Mulvihill (1993) for the National Council for the Elderly.

In some other countries, at least until recently, policy questions about the voluntary sector might have included 'do we have a significant voluntary sector?' or 'do we really need it?'. In Ireland, the questions have revolved more around 'what is the role and contribution of, and justification for, the voluntary sector?', 'how should it be funded?' and 'what should the relationship be between the voluntary and statutory sectors?'. These questions are now looked at in more detail.

Contribution of the voluntary sector

What is the contribution of the voluntary sector to healthcare in Ireland? A surprising point here is that voluntary agencies themselves have not been very effective at articulating their *raison d'être* and their distinctive contribution – some of the larger voluntary agencies could arguably do more to communicate the distinctiveness of their ethos or their contribution to healthcare. It has been left to statutory reports in Ireland in recent years to highlight the contribution of the voluntary sector. According to the Health Strategy, voluntary organisations have been to the forefront in identifying needs and developing responses to them. It refers to their independence and states that they complement statutory services 'in an innovative and flexible manner'.

According to the Commission on Health Funding (1989), the role of voluntary organisations has been immensely important in Ireland. It referred to characteristics such as 'community spirit', 'humanitarianism', 'making available considerable additional resources', identifying and meeting needs quickly, and closeness to client groups.

In general, proponents of voluntary organisations argue that they have a *pioneering/innovative* role, *flexibility* in responding to need, *access* to a large volunteer resource and an opportunity to comment on existing service provision or to act as advocate for their clients. Avan (1986) refers to characteristics such as a questioning of established ways of doing things, risk-taking and a reflection 'with head and heart' on the situations of specific individuals or communities in need. Voluntary organisations also have a specific *educational role*, which facilitates participation in social and political life: for example, increasing public awareness of a disease (educating the public); or developing expertise in how to apply for a grant (educating members).

Philosophical justification for the voluntary sector

Discussion of the practical advantages of the voluntary sector is one thing, but what of the philosophical case for a voluntary sector? The acceptance of the voluntary sector in public discussion can sometimes appear quite pragmatic. In other words, it sometimes appears (as in the work of Johnson) to reflect a perspective about the regrettable limits of the role of the state rather than enthusiasm for the voluntary sector *per se*. The argument is that a comprehensive statutory service can no longer be afforded in many areas, so one has to manage as best one can with the voluntary sector.

Free-market thinking presents a robust critique of a dominant state sector, but does not always provide a strong philosophical justification for the voluntary sector. Free-market writers are philosophically committed to reducing the role, as well as the cost, of the state, on a platform of maximising individual choices. However, proponents of market solutions such as Green (1986) emphasise the rights of private 'for-profit' organisations and autonomous consumers more than what the Americans call 'not-for-profit' organisations.

A more communitarian critique of the state and an implicit justification for voluntary organisations can be found in the work of MacIntyre (1985), who contrasts the politics of the nation state (what he calls the public interest) with the politics of the common good. For the politics of the common good to exist, he says, small societies are necessary, such as co-operatives where people know each other through a web of interactions and there is trust in others and genuine participation in the local community. The politics of the common good, according to MacIntyre, is always the politics of some local community.

In MacIntyre's terms, one model (the common good model)

would be the people of a particular area working out together the health services they require. In the public interest approach, by contrast, the agencies of the State effectively decide the level of health provision in every area.

MacIntyre argues that in the public interest model there is local subordination to central government and that local standards in relation to the common good give way to rational national standards of the public interest. A counter-argument here would be that the political representatives of the people, at both national and regional level, are in fact involved in decision-making about health services, for example through political representatives on Health Boards. Nevertheless, the growth of the consumer movement in public services gives some credence to the analysis of MacIntyre in the sense that it can be seen as a response to perceived inadequacies in the operation of state services, or in the links between those who organise and provide and those who receive services.

A more specific philosophical justification for a flourishing voluntary sector can be found in the principle of 'subsidiarity' – originally advocated by the Catholic Church – which defends the freedom of individuals and smaller groupings to operate and to take initiatives. A Catholic document in the 1930s, *Quadragesimo Anno*, originally defined subsidiarity as follows: 'It is an injustice... to assign to a greater and higher association what lesser and subordinate organizations can do' (par. 79). This principle later inspired E.F. Schumacher (1974), the English author of *Small is Beautiful*.

A more recent Church document, *Instruction on Christian Freedom and Liberation* (Congregation for the Doctrine of the Faith, 1986), stated, in relation to subsidiarity, that 'neither the state nor any society must ever substitute itself for the initiative and responsibility of individuals and of intermediate communities at the level on which they can function, nor must they take away the room necessary for their freedom' (par. 73). Under this definition, subsidiarity is presented as a concept designed to protect personal freedom and initiative and to set limits for state intervention, without denying an important role for the state. Thus the Church – for example, in a recent speech by Archbishop Connell (1996) at the Mater Hospital – has referred to the principle of subsidiarity in its defence of the rights of publicly funded Catholic hospitals against a perceived risk of encroachment by the state.

As well as providing a philosophical justification for the voluntary sector, the Catholic Church has been a major presence in that sector in practice. However, the impact of falling vocations means that that presence is now decreasing.

The principle of subsidiarity has been criticised in Ireland in recent decades, particularly for its espousal of what was seen as an overly negative view of the state. It was criticised, for example, for its justification of Church opposition in 1951 to the 'Mother and Child Scheme' – Dr Noel Browne's unsuccessful attempt to introduce a free universal mother and child health service. This episode has been thoroughly documented, notably by Whyte (1980), but Church concern in Ireland about an increasing role of the state should also perhaps be seen in the context of the expansion of totalitarian regimes in Europe in the 1930s and 1940s.

Circumstances have changed since the 1950s. Church documents today continue to emphasise the principle of subsidiarity, but give equal emphasis to another basic Catholic principle – *solidarity*. In Christian Freedom and Liberation, for example, solidarity is defined as the obligation of persons to contribute to the common good, and is said to reflect Church opposition to social or political individualism. Opposition to collectivism is reflected in the commitment to subsidiarity.

Subsidiarity (on an international rather than a national scale) has also grown in influence in the European Community, for example through the Treaty on European Union (Maastricht Treaty) (European Communities, 1992). This Treaty emphasises that the European Community shall take action only on areas with which the Member States cannot adequately deal on their own: 'In areas which do not fall within its exclusive competence, the Community shall take action, in accordance with the principle of subsidiarity, only if and in so far as the objectives of the proposed action cannot be sufficiently achieved by the Member States and can therefore, by reason of the scale or effects of the proposed action, be better achieved by the Community' (Article 3b).

In summary, the crisis of the Welfare State can be seen as a negative justification for the voluntary sector. The basic positive justification for voluntary organisations is that they meet the needs of service users in a flexible and effective way. An important positive argument in principle for a strong voluntary sector can also be found in the principle of subsidiarity, which has become influential in recent decades. This principle affirms the right of organisations other than the state (or in the case of Europe, the union of states) to exist, to take initiatives and to contribute to the well-being of society. Subsidiarity is an important principle which draws attention to the important role played in civil society both by voluntary organisations and by individuals who take initiatives in contributing to the voluntary sector; and to the need for such organisations and individuals to enjoy the freedom to take appropriate initiatives. It is of interest in this context that an international symposium described by Currin (1992) dealing with former totalitarian regimes in Eastern Europe and South Africa emphasised the contribution of voluntary organisations to democracy and development. The theme of partnership also recurs here. Currin argued that the state was beginning to understand the crucial role that voluntary organisations have to play in development; he also emphasised the importance of a healthy relationship between the voluntary sector and the state.

Issues in statutory–voluntary relationships: obstacles to partnership

The previous section examined actual or potential strengths of the voluntary sector and the philosophical justification for that sector. It is also important to consider problems or issues in the voluntary sector and in the operation of statutory–voluntary relationships – to consider issues which need to be dealt with if the concept of partnership is to become a reality. Some of these problems and issues are set out below. Issues are presented first from the perspective of statutory organisations, and then from the perspective of voluntary organisations.

Statutory concerns

In their comments on statutory–voluntary relationships, statutory organisations often express concern both about *standards* in the voluntary sector and about *reporting relationships* – in other words, about how well voluntary organisations carry out their activities and how well they report such activities.

The Commission on Health Funding gave voice to this concern in 1989 when it argued that difficulties for statutory bodies arise because reporting relationships and standards of accountability appropriate to the provision of public funding have not been laid down for voluntary organisations.

Some of these issues were also highlighted by Midland Health Board personnel in research published by the present author (O'Sullivan, 1994). A problem from the board's point of view was variations in standards between voluntary organisations and the difficulty of monitoring standards (the voluntary view here was that high standards depended largely on adequate levels of funding, and that standards can be just as much an issue in statutory as in voluntary organisations). From the statutory perspective, flexible contracts would be useful in that they would enable the board, in negotiation with the voluntary organisations, to identify and fund appropriate levels of service. At the moment, it was felt, voluntary organisations could have a 'pick and choose' approach, which permitted them not to select certain types of client.

A concern here is that of *comprehensiveness* – in other words, that services provided by the voluntary sector may lack the comprehensiveness of a state-run service; or that if the state is not willing to provide certain services, voluntary organisations may end up carrying out tasks which could more appropriately be carried out by the state. The issue of a lack of comprehensiveness was highlighted, for example, by the Commission on Health Funding (1989)

Another statutory concern, which is related to those already discussed, is that of *co-ordination* of services. If statutory bodies are not clear about what voluntary agencies are doing or if there are issues related to comprehensiveness, then co-ordination of services becomes more difficult.

The co-ordination issue has been highlighted in major national reports. The Health Strategy stated in 1994 that the direct funding of some voluntary agencies by the Department of Health impeded the proper co-ordination of services at local level. The Commission on Health Funding argued that there was a need for a formal framework for the statutory–voluntary relationship – what we might call here a 'structured partnership'. From a statutory perspective, reform of statutory–voluntary relationships has the aim of reducing duplication of services and improving comprehensiveness, by ensuring better co-ordination between the voluntary and statutory services.

Voluntary concerns

From a voluntary perspective, the *discretionary nature of the funding* which voluntary organisations receive is perceived as a problem. The basis for the funding of many voluntary organisations by Health Boards is Section 65 of the Health Act 1953, which allows the funding of organisations providing services 'similar or ancillary' to those provided by the statutory bodies, and Section 26 of the Health Act 1970, which allows Health Boards to arrange for services to be carried out on their behalf. (Some larger providers have been funded directly up to now by the Department of Health. A large mental handicap service agency may indeed receive funding from the Department of Health and the local Health Board and supplementary sources of funding, such as the National Lottery.) In research in the Midlands published by the present author (O'Sullivan, 1994), the Section 65 funding system was described as unsatisfactory by some of those interviewed on the voluntary side. In this perspective, a key problem with Section 65 funding was that the pay side was not treated as pay – that is, if there were national pay increases, health boards did not get these automatically from the Department of Health to cover increases in the pay of staff in voluntary organisations. Yet pay scales in voluntary organisations are linked to those in the health services generally. Delays in Health Board payments were also seen as a problem on the voluntary side.

Issues related to *autonomy* are also of concern to voluntary organisations. Faughnan and Kelleher (1993) reported considerable ambivalence among the voluntary organisations they surveyed about formal contractual arrangements with statutory bodies. This ambivalence was influenced by a feeling that contractual arrangements would affect the capacity of the voluntary organisations to act in an autonomous and innovative manner. Mulvihill (1993) argued, however, that voluntary organisations were open to 'sound contractual arrangements' but that they also stressed the need for consultation on policy, planning, implementation and evaluation.

Lack of influence on planning and policy-making is a significant concern of the voluntary sector. Some of the voluntary organisation personnel interviewed by the author (O'Sullivan, 1994) argued that regional committees in the mental handicap area were not working very effectively. In one view, rather than planning services in a serious way – looking at standards of service, at deficiencies, at whether the right services were being provided, at the allocation within the region of new services – such committees tended to be talking shops.

Writing about care of the elderly, Mulvihill (1993) argued that Health Boards had not adopted the developmental role recommended in *The Years Ahead* (1988) and that few voluntary organisations had any involvement in planning and policy-making. Of the more than 900 voluntary organisations which responded to his study, only about 10% reported any such involvement, and half of this group were not very involved with Health Boards.

In summary, a key aspiration of voluntary organisations is that as movement takes place towards more formal structured relationships with the state, these relationships will be informed by a spirit of genuine partnership and not one of state control.

Current developments – paths to partnership

In response to some of the difficulties and concerns outlined above, several useful new approaches and developments are being advocated in statutory–voluntary relations. Some of these are set out below.

On the voluntary side, there has been concern about the often discretionary nature of the funding which voluntary organisations receive. One significant approach here is to try to define *core* services provided by voluntary organisations which would receive adequate guaranteed funding by state organisations. A National Council for the Elderly report by Lundstrom and McKeown (1994) on home help services for elderly people, for example, argued that this service should be a core service. Core services might then be identified in the contracts between statutory and voluntary agencies, which are discussed below.

In order to create meaningful partnership arrangements, there is considerable interest in creating *effective structures* for statutory–voluntary relations or in rendering more effective existing structures such as the regional committees for the mental handicapped, which bring together statutory and voluntary organisations. As noted above, research carried out by the present author some years ago suggested that there were some problems in the operation of these committees, for example that they were not fulfilling an adequate planning role. In 1997, however, the Department of Health developed a new agreement, *Enhancing the Partnership*, in the disability area.

Supporting Voluntary Activity (1997), the Green Paper on the voluntary and community sector, recommends the strengthening of support structures for the voluntary sector through, for example,

establishing Voluntary Activity Units in certain Government Departments with a responsibility for liaising with voluntary organisations
and establishing a National Support and Development Unit in order
to enhance the infrastructure of support for voluntary activities and
community development (4.14).

There is also a growing interest in funding on a more contractual
basis, through the establishment of *contracts* or *service agreements* between
the statutory and voluntary sectors. Contracts and service agreements
both imply a process setting out what outcomes are expected in return
for the funding provided, and how and when the outcomes will be
measured. The concept of contracting has limitations which are
discussed by Deakin (1996, p. 24) – for example, narrow costs
considerations may prevail in the establishment of contracts, complex
measurement issues may be played down, and voluntary organisations
may be 'weighed down by heavy burdens of bureaucratic requirements
imposed by funding agencies'. Although the terms are closely related,
'service agreement' is perhaps a more suitable term than 'contract'
as it implies a process of collaboration leading to agreement on
services to be provided. Using both service agreement and contracting
terminology, the Commission on Health Funding recommended that
the grant-aid to each voluntary organisation in each area should be
related to the provision of a specific agreed level and type of service;
that the relationship between statutory and voluntary services should
be set out; and that an agreed basis for the evaluation of each agency's
contribution should be developed. This approach, it said, effectively
implied a contractual arrangement 'since funding would be on the
basis of clear agreement on the services to be provided in return'
(par 17.39). Reports in the Southern (1992) and Eastern Health
Boards (1991) recommended contract arrangements between the
Health Board and voluntary agencies. The SHB report argued that
in general grants should not exceed 75% of the cost of a service.

Supporting Voluntary Activity (1997, 4.54) argued that a set of
standard rules in relation to financial accountability should be applied
by all statutory agencies.

As noted above, the Health Strategy was critical of the direct
funding of some large voluntary services by the Department of Health.
In future, it decided, voluntary agencies will receive funding from
the health authorities, to which they will be accountable for the public
funds they have received. A concern of voluntary organisations on

this issue is that there should be a 'level playing field' – in other words, that they will receive the same treatment as the hospitals or other services traditionally run by the Health Boards. Voluntary mental handicap agencies have expressed concern about whether their services will continue to receive priority under new funding arrangements. However, *Enhancing the Partnership* (Working Group on the Implementation of the Health Strategy in relation to Persons with a Mental Handicap, 1997), a new agreement between the Department, the Health Boards and the voluntary agencies, provided reassurance on this point.

The Strategy emphasised that the independent identity of the voluntary agencies would be fully respected under the new structure. They would retain their operational autonomy but would be fully accountable for the public funds which they received. They would continue to have a direct input to the overall development of policy at national level.

The Health Strategy decided that the larger voluntary agencies would have *service agreements* with the health authorities which would link funding by the authorities to agreed levels of service to be provided by the agencies. Agreements would be for a number of years, but the precise level of funding, and the associated service requirements, would be determined annually between the authorities and the agencies concerned. There would be simplified arrangements for smaller groups.

The recommendations of the Health Strategy are now being taken further through the implementation of fundamental change in the healthcare system. In November 1996, the Minister for Health announced that a new Eastern Regional Health Authority would replace the Eastern Health Board and would have responsibility for the funding of all statutory and voluntary services in the region. A task force is currently overseeing the implementation of the reorganisation plans in the East. The Minister also announced that under new legislation, voluntary hospitals, mental handicap agencies and other voluntary agencies would be funded by each local Health Board, rather than by the Department of Health.

Enhancing the Partnership (1997) recommended the establishment of service agreements, an agreed planning framework, and the development of high-quality data, such as those available in the National Mental Handicap Database. It recommended that service agreements be based on key principles, such as the 'rights of persons with mental handicap to quality services which respect their dignity, are provided within the least restrictive environment and aim at the greatest possible inclusion of persons with a mental handicap in society' (p. 26).

Conclusion

This chapter has referred to a growing international interest in the voluntary sector. This interest has a partly negative justification related to the crisis of the Welfare State. The argument in this chapter has been that the positive case for a strong voluntary sector – to be found, for example, in the principle of subsidiarity – and for effective partnership arrangements between statutory and voluntary agencies should also be stressed. Voluntary agencies themselves have an important role to play in communicating their distinctive ethos and contribution to health and social care.

Reference has been made in this chapter to the great diversity of the voluntary sector in Ireland. This diversity makes generalisation difficult, and makes any highly prescriptive approach to partnership arrangements between the statutory and voluntary sectors unwise.

Fundamental changes have taken place or are shortly to take place in the voluntary sector in Ireland and in statutory relationships with the voluntary sector. These include the publication of the Green Paper on the voluntary and community sector; the proposed funding of all voluntary agencies in the East by the Eastern Health Authority, and the development of similar mechanisms in other regions; and a reduced Church presence in the voluntary sector, due to the decline in religious vocations and to changes in the priorities of Catholic agencies.

Changes in funding arrangements and structures, particularly in the Eastern region, where many of the large voluntary agencies are located, will take time to be implemented and to be assessed. Concerns about funding relationships have been expressed in recent times by both sides of the statutory–voluntary partnership. On the statutory side, concerns are sometimes expressed about lack of accountability and value for money in the provision of services by voluntary organisations. On the voluntary side, concerns have been expressed about a possible loss of autonomy in the future, and about the lack of involvement of voluntary organisations in planning and policy-making. Concerns have also been expressed about the impli-cations for mental handicap services of a change to regional from national funding, but a new agreement, *Enhancing the Partnership*, has been worked out in this area.

The argument in this chapter has been that there is a need for a strong voluntary as well as a strong statutory sector in the health services and also for properly structured partnership links between the state and the voluntary sector along the lines of those recommended in some key reports of recent years. There is a need, in other words, for new and more structured relationships in which, as the Health Strategy envisaged, voluntary organisations will retain their autonomy within the context of more adequate structures. On this point, service agreements appear to represent a very fruitful direction in which to proceed, provided that they are not seen mainly as a mechanism of control operating in the interests of the statutory organisation. It is encouraging to note in this context that an SHB report, *A Framework for Caring*, called for increased involvement by voluntary organisations in planning. Voluntary organisations seem ready to accept the development of formal service agreements, but ask in return for adequate *consultation* with the voluntary sector and for significant involvement by voluntary organisations in *planning and policy-making*. Mutually acceptable forms of service agreement need to be worked out in each sector, with the needs of the service user as their point of departure.

This chapter has argued that voluntary–statutory links or structures are extremely important and in need of reform, but it might be added in conclusion that they should also be viewed with realism. In a complex democratic society where needs and organisations change continuously, there will always be a degree of untidiness and imperfection in statutory–voluntary relationships. This means (among other things) that structures, as well as being well-conceived and flexible, must be subject to regular review.

Finally, comment on the voluntary sector has sometimes appeared to assume that, in the future or in an ideal world, all services will come under the statutory umbrella. I have attempted to argue in this chapter that a strong voluntary sector should not be seen as a 'second-best' solution – one imposed on the state, for example, by its fiscal problems – but rather as a very positive reality and resource and a key strength in our tradition of health service provision in Ireland.

CHAPTER 13

Managing Social Services

David Kenefick

Introduction

Social services are provided to a diverse range of client groups including children and adolescents, elderly people, people with disabilities, people with mental health difficulties. As services become more sophisticated and the needs and marginalised position of people in other groups are recognised, social services are also being increasingly provided to travellers, homeless people, people who have substance abuse and addiction problems, and people who are long-term unemployed.

The range of services included under the terms 'social services' and 'social care' is very wide. It includes child protection, family support, enabling people to live independently, helping people to maintain or acquire skills, therapeutic interventions and the provision of a wide range of respite and residential services.

In Ireland, such services are usually provided under the umbrella term of 'health', most of the funding for them comes from the national health budget, and many social services are provided by Health Boards. This, and the fact that there must be considerable co-operation with health services in order to meet some of the needs of the users of social services, contributes to a lack of differentiation between the two types of services and a failure to appreciate fully the need for somewhat different management approaches and practices in social services.

This chapter will look at a number of models which have operated in the social care field and examine those now predominating. It will identify the essential features of a client-centred, community service and will examine some of the implications for managers working to provide such a service.

Models of social care

The charity model

From the eighteenth century onwards this model predominated in many areas of social care, with religious orders and other dedicated people organising and running services for children, people with disabilities and elderly people (Robins, 1980). The legacy of the charity model is seen in the many voluntary groups which provide services to people in these and other groups (McCormack, 1988). This model identified the service receiver (rather than the service user) as needy in some way, and it was the religious or social vocation of the service provider to meet those needs according to the philosophy of their religious order or their social class. This model often merged with another widespread model of social care – the institutional model.

The institutional model

For most of this century this has been the predominant model in services for people with mental health difficulties, and a significant model in services for people with disabilities, children and adolescents. Until 1968, it was the only model of residential care for elderly people (Department of Health, 1988).

The institutional model of managing social care separated the patients from the rest of society and provided a service to them according to centrally devised and administered plans. There was a focus on meeting the basic needs for food, shelter and warmth. Higher level needs for esteem or self-actualisation were rarely acknowledged, much less met (Maslow, 1954). Staff were organised in a hierarchical manner and, in theory at least, all decisions other than the routine were made at a senior level.

This model is still in operation in social care services today. Many institutions remain: the Working Paper on Health Services for the Commission on the Status of People with Disabilities (1996a) points out that the 'psychiatric hospital is still the focal point of the psychiatric service in most parts of the country'.

The model also persists through the training of nurses, doctors and other staff in hospital and other institutions. While placements and other experience of community services have increased considerably, training programmes for doctors and nurses are hospital-based and this has a significant effect on the culture and the practices

199

of those professions (Harrison, 1993).

The institutional model is closely bound up with the medical model.

The medical model

This model derives from a concern with the clinical condition or the pathology underlying the person's condition. This might be evident in a focus on the neurological aspects of an elderly person's deterioration, a teenager's learning disability or a child's very active behaviour. More widely, the medical model uses notions of deficiency or pathology to describe family and social difficulties (Gilligan, 1991).

The Working Paper on Health Services for the Commission on the Status of People with Disabilities (1996a) identifies a major problem with this model. 'The medical model by its nature precludes hope or expectation of recovery or a person's ability to take progressive charge of their own life.' The report goes on to identify the widening of the medical model into the clinical model, involving psychologists and other professionals. According to Barnes (1992) and Oliver (1990), this approach has defined people with disabilities (including mental health difficulties) in terms of some physical, psychological, theological or educational deficit.

Despite its continuing strength in the Irish system, the medical/ clinical model no longer holds absolute sway. Consumers are challenging the power of the clinicians and asserting their own rights.

The community care model

This is the favoured model in social care in Ireland today for all service user groups. Reports on a range of service users (Department of Health, 1988, 1990, 1992a) all support a predominantly community-based approach, with the provision of a range of services in community settings. The National Health Strategy, *Shaping a Healthier Future* (1994), makes it clear that this is government policy for the development of social services.

The community care model means that care and other social services are, to the greatest extent possible, delivered in the community. It is built on the idea of having a mix of services provided by the families of service users, voluntary organisations and statutory agencies co-operating with each other. The complexity of this approach to service provision compared with institutional services is immediately clear. This complexity contributes to the richness of the options and alternatives available to service users, but it also contributes to confusion on their part (Commission on the Status of People with Disabilities, 1996a, 1996b), to overlaps and gaps in service provision, and to a situation in which different agencies have different, and sometimes incompatible, aims for the same client groups (McDaid, 1988).

Two themes may be identified within the community care model: normalisation, and a focus on the rights and dignity of the service users. It is useful to explore each of these themes in some detail.

Normalisation

Wolfensberger (1972), the prime exponent of normalisation, defines it as 'utilisation of means which are as culturally normative as possible, in order to establish and/or maintain personal behaviours and characteristics which are as culturally normative as possible' (p. 28). Put simply, this means enabling people with disabilities and difficulties to live as normally as possible. What is normal is defined partly by society – what behaviours and differences it values – and partly by the professionals who plan, organise and deliver the services. The normalisation approach began to have an impact in Ireland in the 1970s, through the work of professionals in services for people with learning disabilities and people with mental health difficulties, and especially through the use of the PASS (Wolfensberger & Glen, 1975) and PASSING (Wolfensberger & Thomas, 1981) evaluation systems.

The use of the normalisation approach produced many improvements in services: changes from providing places to live in hospitals and institutions to housing in the community, and from care to education and training, are two examples. The normalisation approach still has considerable impact, especially in services for people with mental health difficulties. However, the model has some weaknesses. While it aims for the best for the service users, the best is defined in terms set out by the professionals and by the levels of tolerance of society. The educative focus is on changing people who are different rather than educating society to accept difference. The normalisation approach is being increasingly challenged by a focus on the rights and dignity of service users.

Rights and dignity

This approach to the provision of social services comes from service users themselves expressing their wishes, demanding their rights and demanding respect for difference. They are no longer prepared to accept charity, to be described as patients and dictated to by doctors, or to be normalised by well-meaning professionals (Epstein, 1990; National Economic and Social Forum, 1995; *Report of the Task Force on the Travelling Community*, 1995; Commission on the Status of People with Disabilities, 1996b).

Two short examples will serve to illustrate this model.

1. When the present author taught in a school for young deaf children in the early 1970s, the approach in the school was entirely oral. Children were taught to speak and lip-read English. Signing by pupils, teachers and care staff was forbidden. At the end of primary school those pupils identified as more able continued in an oral stream, while pupils seen as weaker began to learn sign. Today many deaf people see sign as their primary language and part of their cultural identity, which they assert strongly (Matthews, 1996), and there are lively debates within the deaf community about the use of Irish Sign Language versus the use of signed English.

2. Not very long ago, McCormack (1988) could say that society's focus for people with disabilities was a charitable one. More recently, the *Irish Times* (7 January 1997) could make strong, unqualified statements in a leading article:

   > ...most of the handicaps faced by people with disabilities are social, not medical. If people with disabilities cannot use public transport it is not the fault of their disabilities, it is the fault of CIE. If people with disabilities cannot get into a hotel, it is the fault of the hotel, not the fault of their disabilities. If people with disabilities cannot get job interviews, it is the fault of those who select candidates, not the fault of their disabilities.

Client-centred care: the aims and benefits

At the core of the community care model is the belief in client-centred or person-centred care. The primacy of the consumer is strongly emphasised in *Shaping a Healthier Future* (1994). This has a particular significance for the social services, which are concerned with very broad aspects of people's lives such as where they live or how safe they are.

Shaping a Healthier Future did not introduce the notion of client-centred care in the community. This idea already existed in Irish social services and, as noted above, was endorsed by reports on a number of sectors (Department of Health, 1988, 1990, 1992a). What the Health Strategy did was to indicate clearly that this was the appropriate model for all social services, and that this model had government and Departmental backing.

The key aim of the client-centred approach is to place the client, and meeting the client's needs, at the centre of the planning, organisation and delivery of services.

The second aim of client-centred services is that of providing *social gain*. This improvement in the quality of a person's life may be, for example, through the provision of somewhere for them to live safely or through supporting them to take part in educational or leisure activities.

The Strategy states that 'Social gain is concerned with broader aspects of the quality of life'. This definition is very broad and is markedly less precise than the definition of health gain. This lack of precision presents problems in the interpretation of what is meant and in attempts to measure the outcomes of social service interventions.

The third aim of client-centred services is that they should be delivered in the community in the setting which is most appropriate for the individual client. Until this is done, services cannot be said to be truly client-centred, as organisational aspects of the service inevitably take precedence in an institutional setting.

This approach has major benefits for the client, but it also has benefits for the staff and for managers.

For the client:

- the client's needs are more important than the needs of the service
- the client can receive different types and amounts of service when he or she needs them
- the client has more influence over the policies, organisation and delivery of services.

For the staff:

- staff can share responsibility for the quality of services with clients
- frontline staff have much more autonomy and decision-making

power than in an institutional service

- staff can work in ordinary settings, with people from other sectors, and so are less cut off from the rest of life
- there are greater opportunities for job development and enrichment as services change and develop to meet client needs.

For the manager:

- the manager can use resources flexibly and creatively to meet client needs rather than simply allocating them to units or places
- there are many opportunities for the manager to innovate and to pilot new types of service
- he or she can have more autonomy earlier in her/his career than would be possible in an institutional setting
- the manager can spend more time in ordinary settings working with people from other sectors to ensure that the needs of her/ his clients are met.

How can a service be client-centred?

In order to put the client at the core of the service, a number of things must happen.

- The needs of the client must be the primary factor in how services are organised and delivered, rather than the structure and organisation of the services or the way in which funding is allocated.
- The client must be consulted about the type and extent of services to be provided to them.
- The client must have a choice about the kind of service which they need at any point in time.
- The client must be involved in decisions about the policies and organisation of the service.
- The client must be able to access different types of services provided by different departments and agencies without having to go through complicated referral and assessment procedures.
- Services must respond flexibly to the changing needs of the individual client.
- Services should be delivered in the most appropriate setting for the individual client rather than in settings that are the easiest to administer or most convenient for the professionals involved.

In summary, services should be decentralised, flexible, responsive to clients' needs and multi-agency, and should involve high levels of client consultation and participation (Commission on the Status of People with Disabilities, 1996b).

Most social services are still in transition from institutional and organisation-centred models to a client-centred, community model (not always successfully, as both McGowan (1996) and Brown (1996) point out). For managers, this often means working to achieve aims set within the context of the client-centred model using procedures designed for an institutional model.

Many managers of social services are struggling to facilitate the transition from institution to community. They are aided by the expressed wishes of clients, the aims set out in *Shaping a Healthier Future*, and the approach of many social service staff. They are hindered by many of the organisational, financial and accountability arrangements, by the way in which many staff are trained, by the transfer of institutional thinking and practices into the community, and by the tensions between the felt needs of clients and the needs and wishes of families and communities.

Issues in managing a client-centred community service

Balance between client and other needs

In delivering a social service, an agency or an individual professional is rarely working exclusively with a single individual. The primary client usually has family members who are concerned about the client's welfare, have their own views about how this should be safeguarded, and also have their own needs. Mittler and Mittler (1994, p. 8) stress that '...the needs of the individual should never be considered in isolation from the social, family and political context in which they are embedded'. Local communities, consumer groups and even the state may also claim a stake in decision-making.

Service providers must have ways of distinguishing between the different sets of needs, prioritising them and, if it is appropriate, meeting them separately. In some cases significant needs of the primary client may be obscured by the way the situation is described by relatives. Thus, for example, an elderly person may want to continue to live alone with support. The person's relatives may feel that the situation is too risky and too demanding of their time and attention, so they present the need for a residential place.

While social services have a responsibility to the primary client, the family and others in such situations, an underlying principle should be that clients are not placed in more restrictive situations simply to meet the needs of relatives or assuage the fears of communities. There is increased danger of this happening in situations where staff are working under great pressure and have limited resources for working with family members to help them to allow their relative to make his or her own choices.

Consultation and participation

The importance of these two processes cannot be overemphasised. A key difference of social services from health services is that clients are often involved with social services for very long periods of time. They therefore have an interest in how the services are planned and managed in a way that those who have only brief contact with a service do not.

Some of the ways in which individual clients can and should be involved in the planning and organisation of social services delivered to them are as follows.

- *Identifying client needs* (Fiedler and Twitchin, 1992). Clients have a different point of view on their needs from both the service providers and other family members, and this should be reflected in the process. Defining service needs in terms of what a client wants to be able to do, rather than in terms of what services are available, is a significant step in making services client-centred rather than agency-centred.
- *Making/participating in decisions about the nature and extent of services they will receive and making choices in their lives.* Fiedler (1993), Deakin & Thomas (1995) and Rafferty (1996) all emphasise the need to give the service user choices in the types of service he or she wants to use, allowing the exercise of options both within services and between service providers.
- *Involvement in decisions about the ongoing management and policies of the service* (National Rehabilitation Board, 1994; Youll & McCourt-Perring, 1993).
- *Involvement in the planning of the service* (Towell, 1988; Welsh Health Planning Forum, 1993).

- *Access to an effective complaints procedure* helps to ensure that standards are maintained and that the need for changes in procedures or staff behaviour are identified (National Economic and Social Forum, 1995; Commission on the Status of People with Disabilities, 1996b).

Steps that managers can take to enable clients to have the types of involvement cited above

The clients

- Give clients information so that they have a real picture of the resources and options available to them (National Economic and Social Forum, 1995).
- Provide support to those clients who need it in order to participate. This may be done through frontline staff and through the development of advocacy and self-advocacy programmes (Sutcliffe & Simons, 1993; Commission on the Status of People with Disabilities, 1995). Managers also need to be aware of special needs of client groups, e.g. particular media, literacy or access needs in planning consultation.
- Move towards having service users as members of policy, planning and review groups as a matter of course (Epstein, 1990; Commission on the Status of People with Disabilities, 1996b).

The organisation

- Start from the premise that it is the right of the client to be involved and that it is the manager's job to find ways of making that happen.
- Encourage the development of a culture in the service which enables clients rather than making them dependent on the professionals and on the service.
- Work to convince senior management and board members of the importance of client consultation and participation.
- Work with staff to ensure that they are convinced of the necessity and advantages of involving service users.
- Support frontline staff in finding and using mechanisms which give clients a real voice in various processes involved in planning, running and reviewing services.
- Help staff to access and use information on experiences in other

services through visits, talks and written reports, remembering that this information will be used only if the manager is committed to the principle of participation.

- Approach complaints as opportunities to communicate with service users and to improve the services rather than as a threat against which they must defend themselves and the service.
- Examine the various procedures used in the agency to ensure that they are readily understood and easily used by clients, and to see whether proper follow-up procedures are in place which ensure improvements in practices (Brechin & Swain, 1987; Handy, 1988; Sutcliffe & Simons, 1993; Commission on the Status of People with Disabilities, 1996b).

Quality and effectiveness

Quality

Quality in social services may be difficult to define and agree on. Different types of service will have different aims and therefore different ways of defining quality.

Shaping a Healthier Future (Department of Health, 1994) discusses ways of measuring quality in the services but does not specifically define it. The closest it gets to a definition is in describing social gain, which it identifies as the quality added to people's lives as a result of service interventions. One way of describing service quality, then, is in terms of its effectiveness in adding to the quality of people's lives. Definitions of quality are explored more fully in Chapter 10.

One overriding aspect of every service is the quality of the interactions between the staff providing the service and the service users. How staff relate to and treat clients is at the heart of every social service – and this is based not just on their own beliefs and attitudes but on the aims and standards of the service (Brechin & Swain, 1987; College of Speech and Language Therapists, 1991; Joyce & Kenefick, 1997).

Because it is difficult to measure many of the quality aspects of social services, we often fail even to try. *Shaping a Healthier Future* recognises that quality in the health and social services may be difficult to measure, and warns against giving precedence to those features of the service that are easier to measure. Despite this, there is still a tendency to count the number of complaints, to record the number of people seen in a week or to specify the average length of time on a waiting list rather than to try to measure the quality of a staff–client interaction, to identify the extent to which a staff member is promoting a client's independence, or to measure the appropriateness of a particular intervention. This tendency is encouraged by the types of records required by the Department of Health, which, while it advocates the measurement of outcomes, still requires services to measure inputs.

Most social services are still in transition from institutional and organisation-centred models to a client-centred, community model (not always successfully, as McGowan (1996) and Brown (1996) point out). For managers, this often means working to achieve aims set within the context of the client-centred model using procedures designed for an institutional model.

This chapter is too short to examine ways of measuring quality and effectiveness in any detail, but some simple questions may help to point managers and staff in the right direction.

- What are we trying to achieve?
- Who needs to be involved in order for us to achieve our aims?
- How will we know when we have succeeded?

All these questions should be asked *with* service users.

Maintaining quality when demand is high

Most social service agencies are operating in the context of very high levels of demand for their services. Child protection services have growing numbers of referrals and are unable to undertake the preventive work they wish to do (Barnardos, 1997); services for elderly people are under pressure because of the growing numbers of people requiring services and the increased range of services they want; most areas of the country still do not have nearly enough supported residential accommodation for people with learning disabilities.

At the same time, staff working in these services want to provide a high-quality service. There is a constant tension between the aim of providing a service to as many people as possible and providing an appropriate and high-quality service. These aims are often presented as incompatible opposites. Poor quality of service and lack of consultation with service users are explained away with reference to the numbers of people who are being provided with a service. Social service managers cannot wait for some ideal world in which they will have sufficient resources available to enable them to provide a quality service. They have a responsibility to use the resources available to them now to provide the best possible service to as many as possible of those who need it.

In the situation in which Irish social services are operating, a number of things are critically important for the delivery of quality services (Kieran, 1988; Cullen, 1988; Joyce & Kenefick, 1997):

- agreement on the purpose and aims of each service – this agreement needs to reach from the frontline to the top of the service organisation, and must include the funders
- the involvement of the users of the service in setting the aims and the standards for the service
- the establishment of standards of service – these should be positive standards, not just rules for preventing abuse or accidents
- the provision of training related to the purpose and aims of the service, which meets the immediate training needs of the staff.

Effectiveness

It can be difficult to measure the effectiveness of social services because of a lack of clarity or agreement about the desirable outcomes and because it may be hard to find reliable ways of measuring those outcomes. In a client-centred service, outcomes must be specified in terms of meeting identified client needs. This might mean that the client secures a job, is able to mix with peers without becoming involved in fights, or takes part in chosen social activities. These real outcomes contrast with the more typical descriptions of service to clients, which are really descriptions of inputs. These include the allocation of a community residential place, enrolment in a socialisation programme and so many hours of visits from a social worker.

In setting goals against which to measure effectiveness, it is essential to start with the client. A really good-quality nursing home place provided within one week will not be the best outcome for an elderly person who wants to continue to live in her own home. So, while the service in itself may be of a very good quality, it is not effective in meeting the client's need.

In many cases social care services are provided over a very long period of time, so that it is a question not so much of measuring the quality and effectiveness of a particular episode of treatment or care as of continually monitoring and reviewing both. In such long-term situations there is a wonderful opportunity to develop a real partnership with the service users in ways which are simply not possible for acute services. This may be challenging, even frightening, for staff who are trained and used to making the decisions on their own. Staff need support to develop such relationships (Brechin & Swain, 1987).

Changing non-client-centred resources into a client-centred service

In order to use resources in a client-centred way, it is necessary for managers to understand the needs, to understand the best ways of meeting them, to know what resources are available and to know how these resources can be managed to meet the needs. This is the real reason for understanding financial procedures. A good manager can see how different allocations of money can be combined, how new and creative services can be fitted into existing financial reporting, and where it is possible to stop old ineffective practices in order to fund newer, more client-centred services, and can generate support for these options.

Social services managers with a strong client focus often feel that a focus on budgets is a waste of time. This may be because their experience of budgeting has been entirely negative and restrictive, or because the whole area seems difficult and esoteric. However, if managers with this strong client focus want to ensure that that focus is the predominant one in their organisation, they do need to pay attention to money and how they can best use it for their clients. For most managers this means that they need training so that they can talk to finance staff on an equal footing and so that they can challenge some of the accepted wisdom in their organisation about how money is allocated and accounted for. In order to make an organisation client-focused it is necessary to learn to use financial resources well and to inform those with special responsibility for finance about the needs of clients.

Supporting and protecting staff

Work in social services can be stressful and pressurised: clients may be suffering trauma, may be demanding, aggressive or difficult to communicate with; waiting lists for service may be long with resulting crises and queries from families, other agencies and politicians; the public may be demanding service for your client group, but not near where they themselves live (Doherty, 1996). Support by a manager for her/his staff must be real and practical, not just aspirational or on paper. Ways of providing real support include:

- working to develop a good local team in which staff work co-operatively and support each other
- meeting individual frontline staff, both formally and informally – these contacts allow a manager to learn more about the qualities of individual staff, the needs on the ground and possible improvements to the service
- attending staff meetings regularly and hearing about successes and difficulties
- providing information to staff on levels of need, current and future funding, organisational plans, training and development opportunities, and research and new practice in the field
- paying attention to the needs for physical resources, learning to distinguish between those which are essential and those which are not, and working very hard to provide the essential requirements
- providing short-term extra resources (even if this means cutting back later) in a crisis situation – these could include extra staff, additional input from clinical advisers, additional equipment
- the manager being an ambassador for her/his staff – this means telling senior management about the successes of the team, the pressures they are under and the impact on them of organisational decisions; a good manager keeps her/his staff in mind when discussing changes and developments
- celebrating success in a visible way – how this is done will depend on the scale of the success and the circumstances, but the manager should not be inhibited by an organisational culture which does not celebrate success; she or he can start a change in the culture
- ensuring that frontline staff have communication routes other than through their immediate manager to ensure that bad practices by a frontline manager do not do irreparable damage to a team.

Multi-agency delivery of services - developing relationships with other agencies

Social services in Ireland are delivered by a range of statutory and voluntary bodies which come under a number of broad headings, including health, social welfare, local government, community development, employment and education. The individual needs of clients can more easily be met if these different agencies develop shared aims and objectives, co-operate, share information and resources. Within the social services field, co-operation between statutory and voluntary agencies is critical. Services are delivered to most client groups by a mixture of both types of service, and lack of co-operation or, worse still, competition can only have an adverse effect on services to clients.

It is important for managers to be aware of the enormous advantages which may accrue to their clients from co-operation between agencies, and of the imperative in the National Health Strategy for co-operation. For clients to gain these advantages, however, they must be assisted in finding their way through the maze of different services to those which they want. (Browne, 1992; Commission on the Status of People with Disabilities, 1996b; *Report of the Task Force on the Travelling Community*, 1995).

Delivering a decentralised service

In order to be truly client-centred and community-based, services must be decentralised and delivered in the most appropriate setting for the individual client. Only when services are taken to the clients in their own streets and villages, in their own homes and places of work, in their own shops and clubs, can they truly be said to be client-centred. The client-centred focus demands a shift not just in money and buildings but in models of service delivery and in staff and management roles.

Management approaches and styles need to be different for decentralised services which are provided in people's own homes and workplaces, in foster homes or in small community-based houses from those which are appropriate in single-site hospitals and institutions. The manager of a decentralised community service is managing services which affect where and how people live and work, often balancing client independence with risks to the client, balancing the client's rights with the attitudes of the local community, and even

213

balancing the needs and rights of clients and their carers. This work must be done out in the community without the protection which the institutional setting gives to a manager. It is a demanding job which calls for a different emphasis in the application of management skills and different attitudes to those required for managing a large hospital or institution (Quinn, 1990; Adirondack, 1992; McGowan, 1996).

In the author's experience, there are a number of essential requirements for managing a decentralised community service, as follows.

Presence on the ground:
- spending as much time as possible listening to frontline staff and clients and away from the office and headquarters meetings
- developing relationships with individual clients and with clients' groups
- building links with the local community.

Developing and supporting staff:
- developing the knowledge and skills of first-line managers so that they can manage their own part of the service
- developing understandings with first-line managers which clarify decision-making processes in the organisation and allow the managers to operate more independently
- developing understandings with first-line managers and staff as to what constitutes a crisis or a serious situation which requires the manager's immediate attention
- building a team with professional and administrative colleagues to maximise the input from different disciplines into major decisions
- being ready to step in to support staff and clients in a crisis, even if the support should be coming from someone else
- decentralised community services demand significant staff training and development – the manager's job is to develop the first-line managers reporting to her/him and to help them to develop their staff.

Developing her/his own management skills:
- putting significant effort into prioritising her/his work and managing her/his time and being prepared to deal with phone calls, letters and reports away from the comfort of the office

- developing her/his own skills in delegation
- being able to live with uncertainty and risk in the development of new forms of service and in decisions made regarding individual clients
- accessing real support for herself/himself because of the very high levels of demand on her/him – without real support a manager is in danger of experiencing severe stress and burnout over time.

Systems

Systems for recording and reporting work with clients are essential in ensuring a quality service, in preventing abuse and in appraising staff performance. These systems need to be designed so that they support good work with clients, and not in a way which makes them an end in themselves.

Developing a long-term view

For social services to stay client-centred, it is necessary for managers to develop a long-term view of the needs of clients and potential clients and of ways of meeting these needs. This can be difficult for managers who are constantly under pressure to meet immediate needs, deal with crises or reduce waiting lists. However, if services are to develop, managers need to be constantly looking forward. This means keeping in touch with the thinking of the Department of Health, with research and developments in other countries, with the views of staff on the ground and, most particularly, with consumers. To do this managers must find time to read, attend conferences, visit other services and explore their own thinking about possible futures.

A long-term view also necessitates the development of plans for a number of years ahead. The development of longer term plans is one of the essential activities of management (Covey *et al.*, 1994), but it tends to be neglected in social services, which are so often crisis-driven. There is an imperative for managers to meet the immediate needs of clients and demands of their organisation, the Health Board, the public, politicians, the media! While managers must pay attention to these immediate needs and demands, paying exclusive attention to them will inevitably lead to the development of a crisis culture. Such a culture will have bad outcomes for clients which will have a bad impact on them over a long period of time.

215

Conclusion

This chapter has described some of the main models of social care provision and has explored the currently predominant model and its implications for managers. While many of the skills, qualities and activities described are good management practice in any organisation, they are critical for managers in social services. The potential impact of bad management practices on clients' lives is very significant. Because many clients are involved with social services for long periods of time, such effects are cumulative. Social service managers must be aware that their decisions can have profound effects on the lives of the users of their services. The major way in which they can build and strengthen this awareness is by being closely involved with the clients of the service.

These are demanding times for managers in the social services. Despite, or perhaps because of, increasing prosperity there is a very high level of demand for services; government and consumer both expect quality services; new problems and issues continue to emerge and there is increased scrutiny by the media. They are also exciting times: there are new opportunities for partnerships with service users, for partnerships between organisations and for partnerships between sectors. Managing social services today is a highly skilled and a highly demanding activity, and managers themselves have a role in specifying and developing the skills and in defining and meeting the demands.

PART SIX

Clinicians, Professionals and the Management Process

CHAPTER 14

Doctors and Management Development

Laraine Joyce

Introduction

As doctors have a major responsibility for the way in which resources are used in healthcare, it comes as no surprise that they are increasingly being called upon to become more involved in the management process. Ham & Hunter (1988) identified three main strategies whereby doctors, managers and politicians could seek to promote efficiency and effectiveness in healthcare:

1. raise professional standards through medical audit and accreditation
2. involve doctors in management by providing them with budgets and encouraging them to manage
3. external management control through managing clinical work, changing the contracts of doctors and promoting competition between providers.

Each of these strategies has been used to some extent in Ireland. Leahy *et al.* (1997), for instance, reported on the experiences in introducing surgical audit into three Irish hospitals. They concluded that the three factors most crucial to the success of audit were:

- the commitment of consultants
- the support of management
- having a reliable software product.

Apart from their work and that of a number of others, medical audit and accreditation are relatively underdeveloped in Ireland.

Recent attention has focused on the second and third of the strategies identified by Ham & Hunter (1988), namely the agreement on a new contract for consultants and the promise of initiatives to involve doctors more in the healthcare management process.

Thus, as this chapter was being completed, the negotiations on a new contract for hospital consultants were reaching a conclusion. The recent report of the Review Body on Higher Remuneration in the Public Sector on hospital consultants (1996) expressed strong dismay at the slow rate of progress in involving consultants in a more meaningful way in the hospital management process. It commented that there was a growing interest among consultants in participating in the management of hospitals, and that this opportunity had to be seized. The Review Body noted that 'the key motivation for consultants is to ensure that their management roles offer them real power, influence and responsibility with corresponding accountability'.

The Review Body made a number of recommendations regarding hospital management structures centring on devolving decision-making and budgets within hospitals to units that would operate at sub-board level. These units could be based on specialities, departments, directorates or other appropriate groupings, depending on the hospital's size and role. It recommended that consultants who took on a managerial role should be provided with the appropriate training, support staff and other facilities. If doctors are to make a fuller contribution to the management process within hospitals it is essential, therefore, that they get help and support in developing the necessary competencies.

In this chapter I consider the rationale and the problems associated with involving doctors in management, and the experiences of providing management development for doctors, and outline the results of a recent survey of Irish consultants and senior registrars regarding their perceived management development needs. The chapter concludes with outline recommendations for management development initiatives to prepare the way for a greater involvement by doctors in management within hospitals in Ireland.

Why involve doctors in management?

Disken *et al.* (1990) made a case for involving doctors in management on the basis that it helps to devolve decision-making within hospitals to those responsible for delivering the service – a management principle advocated in the Dublin Hospital Initiative Group reports of 1990 and 1991. It can also serve to break down barriers between doctors, managers and other healthcare professionals. Other perceived benefits that Diskin *et al.* identify include:

- improved clarity of service objectives
- improved quality of planning and higher budgetary control
- decentralised and therefore faster decision-making
- greater flexibility in responding to changing demands.

These benefits should result in a better service for patients. As the Review Body (1996) points out, consultants play a key role in determining, through their clinical decisions, the pay and non-pay costs of hospitals. The pattern of healthcare delivery in the acute sector is primarily determined by the clinical output of consultants' individual practices. They must therefore be part of any process that attempts to improve the efficiency and effectiveness of acute services that absorb so much of health spending.

The ultimate justification for doctors' becoming more involved in the management process is thus that the care to patients will be improved. That is the criterion against which any changes in practice must be judged.

Levels of managerial responsibility

All doctors manage. Even if they do not have a formally designated management role, they nevertheless have to manage their time, their patients, the facilities they use and the staff who report to them.

However, doctors can have varying levels of involvement in the management process (Allen, 1995). At the most basic level (level 1), all doctors have a responsibility to manage their own time, patients and their immediate support staff. At the next level (level 2), doctors may become involved in more general management processes through their participation in management or speciality committees. They thus contribute to management decision-making beyond the remit of their own firm or practice. At the next level of involvement in management (level 3), some consultants may assume responsibility for the delivery of a service, typically in the clinical directorate model where a consultant becomes a clinical director and manages a budget and the delivery of services, supported by a business manager and a nurse manager. In that case, the consultant is acting as a leader on behalf of other consultants who are delivering a service. It would seem that such a model has so far become established in a very small number of

Irish hospitals. At the highest level of involvement (level 4), a consultant may become a medical director, and thereby contribute to the strategic direction and strategic management of the organisation. The Master in a maternity hospital and the Resident Medical Superintendent in a psychiatric hospital are examples. Doctors may also become involved in policy-making in other ways, for instance through their membership of Health Boards.

A difficult role

Doctors who have or will have a significant management responsibility occupy a difficult role. They will need support and encouragement in that role. As they are likely to be caught in a kind of 'no man's land' between management and other doctors, it is not likely that they will find such support in either constituency.

Burgoyne & Lorbiecki (1993) found that a major determinant of whether or not clinicians became involved in management was their desire and need to maintain their credibility with other clinicians. This also determined the speed and form in which they became involved in management.

The consultants whom Burgoyne & Lorbiecki interviewed were becoming involved in formal management roles, usually through clinical directorates. This is how their strategies were described:

> Many of them were very conscious of keeping their 'lines of retreat' open. They viewed and were viewed as an experimental, 'reconnoitre' group, both for themselves and their colleagues, many of whom they described as 'playing a waiting game' themselves before deciding whether to pursue some of the more managerial options. In this sense they could present themselves as exploring the management option on behalf of their colleagues, and in doing so retain their places within the medical culture. (p. 254)

Resistance to a managerial role

Resistance to assuming a managerial role is not uncommon among doctors. Gatrell and White (1996), for instance, found a broad 30:70 split between doctors receptive to a managerial role and those antagonistic to it.

Walker & Morgan (1996) outlined some of the reasons for resistance by the medical profession to a greater involvement. These include a perception that it is not central to their role as a consultant, that it may be at odds with their aim of providing the best possible care to individual patients, and that it may erode their clinical autonomy. It could be said, however, that one doctor's clinical autonomy is another doctor's opportunity cost. Doctors can stand to benefit directly from their personal involvement in management in so far as it enables them to influence the determination of priorities for their particular hospital or service.

Management is also seen as being a role of lower status and standing in the community (Burgoyne & Lorbiecki, 1993). This acts as an additional disincentive to doctors in taking on significant managerial responsibilities.

Doctors who take on a managerial role thus face significant stress. They may have to face difficult dilemmas. Choosing to enhance services for a greater number of patients in the longer term may mean a reduced level of service to presenting patients in the short term. Such choices tend to conflict with medical codes of practice, which emphasise the doctor's responsibility to provide the best possible treatment for each of his or her patients. Becoming involved in formal management is perhaps most difficult for consultants when it means that their managerial role may conflict with the managerial role of their colleagues. This suggests a more hierarchical model than the traditionally flat peer-to-peer relationship between consultants, whereby consultant representatives are usually elected or appointed on a consensual basis.

A study undertaken by Middlesex University found that junior doctors have a poor understanding of the role of the doctor-manager (Newman & Pyne, 1994). They had not been sufficiently prepared for a role in management, but they were nevertheless very positive to the idea of clinicians playing a role in hospital management. They themselves were willing to assume management responsibilities when the time came. This may suggest that future consultants will be more receptive to assuming a managerial role.

However, time constraints can be another difficulty. A 1997 survey of clinical directors in the UK (Simpson & Scott, 1997) found that most were working nearly double their contracted hours on management duties; nearly half felt undervalued for their management contribution and had problems in fulfilling their clinical commitments. Almost half of them were thinking about going back to full-time clinical practice and giving up their managerial role. The authors concluded that:

> While there is evidence of clinical directors taking on a more strategic role, the involvement of doctors in management is still hugely vulnerable and tenuous. The enormous benefits clinical directors can bring to the management of trusts will only be realised with continuing effort by chairs, chief executives and trust boards. (p. 25)

A clash of cultures

Fitzgerald and Sturt (1996) point to the existence of two cultures side by side within hospitals: the medical and the managerial/administrative cultures. Medical culture is seen to contain three elements:

- the professional attitudes and values of clinical autonomy
- the use of specialist language
- specific work practices which can be related to mental habits and orientations.

Clinical freedom is seen as a key aspect of medical culture, particularly in discussions of doctors and their managerial responsibilities. Both the managerial and the medical cultures tend to use specialist language that can impede communication and lead to stereotyping.

While both doctors and managers practise management, the nature of that practice tends to be different (Burgoyne & Lorbiecki, 1993). Doctors are engaged, for the most part, in operational management. They are concerned with the allocation of resources in the short term – with their effects on their individual patients who are currently under treatment – and they tend to make their decisions on their own, in the tradition of clinical autonomy. This contrasts with the collective, long-term, team-based, resource procurement nature of formal management.

Management development for doctors

A conference was convened in Dublin in May 1993 to consider the management development of doctors as managers of clinical resources. Organised under the auspices of the European Healthcare Management Association, it included representatives from ten countries. The conference delegates agreed that changes are under way in healthcare systems in all developed countries and that these will impact heavily on the medical profession. According to Boufford (1994, p. 6):

> The strongest feeling is one of a shifting of power in new directions – from hospital specialists to hospital managers; from hospital-based doctors to general practitioners and other primary care doctors; from doctors to other health professionals; and from doctors to patients. The common denominator is a relative loss of power by all doctors, but especially hospital-based ones, traditionally the most clinically autonomous and managerially independent of the other segments of the healthcare system.

If it is accepted that such a change and a shift of power is under way in Ireland also, then part of the role of management development for doctors should be to enable doctors who are in the middle of the change process to respond.

Allen (1995, p. 47) argues that if a doctor wants to improve the efficiency of services, then an investment in management training will be worth while. As he says:

> Much of management theory is systematised common sense and intelligent people intuitively develop many of the principles for themselves and 'have been doing it all along'. Where a management programme can help is to provide a structure to enable doctors to name what they have often long been doing and to show them that there is a structure which can help them to understand what they have been doing and hopefully manage better. Participating in management programmes provides them with 'jargon'... Another effect is that they become more tolerant of managers, as they gain an insight into the world of management and realise that there may be method in their madness.

Allen concludes that management training aims to enable doctors to do a management job better and also to do a better job generally.

The benefits of management development were also commented on by the consultants interviewed by Burgoyne & Lorbiecki (1993). They found it useful to learn the language of management and to learn that management was not the technically certain exercise they had presumed it to be. This increased their confidence in acting in managerial roles and enabled them to talk to managers in their own terms.

A postal survey was carried out in the UK of medical directors of

NHS trusts (Wood *et al.*, 1995). Their views were sought on their existing managerial knowledge, their training/preparation prior to becoming medical director, and their advice to future medical directors regarding training needs. The areas of knowledge that were deemed to be most essential by medical directors were strategic planning, communication skills, time management, medical ethics and negotiation skills. They felt that future medical directors would benefit most from on-the-job training and specialist training in medical management. MBAs or MScs in public health were not seen as being appropriate. The authors concluded that it was no longer appropriate for senior physicians to undertake a management role without management training.

Gatrell & White (1996) concluded from their study that the management learning needs of doctors are progressive, according to their grade or seniority within the system. Most interesting, perhaps, they found that whereas doctors, and consultants in particular, rated their interpersonal skills very highly, this did not match with the perceptions of those with whom they worked.

Walker & Morgan (1996) advocate a more strategic approach to management development for doctors in Wales, whereby those doctors with an interest in, and an aptitude for, management should be identified. This would then facilitate the planning of individualised management development programmes for them. The authors warn that while considerable amounts of money have been spent in attempting to meet the management development needs of future consultants, this has been done in a relatively haphazard and unstructured way and appeared to have been of little benefit to the recipients.

Burgoyne & Lorbiecki (1993) warn that the long-term success of efforts to involve doctors in management will depend on the extent to which medical culture and the professional self-image of doctors can adapt and change and they can accept the managerial model that other professionals, such as accountants and solicitors, have taken on board.

The situation in Ireland

What is the situation in Ireland? Are consultants indeed showing a growing interest in management, as the Review Body suggested? Are senior registrars more interested in assuming a managerial role? What kinds of management training have our doctors received? What do they perceive their management training needs to be, and how would they like them to be met? Brady (1994) provided a useful overview of management development for doctors in Ireland, but it was deemed useful to try to ascertain the up-to-date position by directly consulting doctors themselves. As the preceding review of literature has indicated, much of the research has been based on the experience in the UK and there is a need to compare and contrast the experience in Ireland and, indeed, to build up a body of research in this area.

Postal survey of Irish consultants and senior registrars

To answer these and other questions, a postal survey was undertaken of Irish consultants and senior registrars. The questionnaire used was based closely on one used in a survey of doctors in the North-Western Regional Health Authority in the UK (Horsley *et al.*, 1996) to allow comparison of responses across the two systems.

Questionnaires were posted to all consultants listed in the *Irish Medical Directory* and to all senior registrars (based on a listing provided by the Postgraduate Medical and Dental Board) in February/March 1997. In all, 1141 consultants and 270 senior registrars were sent a questionnaire. A response rate of 24% was obtained from consultants and 32% from senior registrars. This compares with a UK response rate of 68% in 1994 and 48% in 1987 (in a previous survey). Horsley *et al.* (1996) attributed their increase in response from 1987 to 1994 to the fact that reminder letters were sent out in 1994 but not in 1987. Walker & Morgan (1996) achieved a response rate of over 50% in a survey they conducted of consultants and senior registrars in the NHS in Wales, while Gatrell & White (1996) achieved a 30% response rate in England. No reminder letters were sent to the Irish doctors. The specialities most likely to respond in Ireland were accident and emergency, medicine and paediatrics. The lowest response rates were from consultants in anaesthesia, pathology, obstetrics and gynaecology.

In Ireland, the consultants who responded reflected the age distribution of the general population of consultants. Thus, 12% were between 30 and 39 years of age, 50% in their forties and the remainder over 50. All the senior registrars were in their thirties. As regards gender, 12% of the consultants were female, as compared to 18% of the senior registrars. Women held 18% of permanent consultant posts in 1997, so one would have expected a slightly higher response rate from the female consultants.

227

Management responsibilities

All consultants have management responsibility for themselves, their patients and their immediate staff. Of the consultants who responded to the survey, 54% said they had management responsibility for areas in addition to these. This group with additional management responsibilities was not significantly different from the rest of the sample in terms of either age or gender. Somewhat surprisingly, the corresponding figure from the UK survey was lower at 47%.

An examination of the Irish responses revealed that consultants reported they held a wide range of management responsibilities. These included being chairman or secretary to the medical board or to a speciality committee. Consultants also reported that they had responsibilities as a director, for example, of radiology, accident & emergency (A & E), etc. Others were members of the board of the hospital or had significant teaching responsibilities. Several of the respondents who stated that they had no additional managerial responsibilities responded in terms that indicated that they saw their primary responsibility as being for the treatment of patients – that was what they became a doctor to do – and that they had no interest in management, but left that to the 'administrators'.

Of the Irish consultants who said they had additional management responsibility, only 15% said they received any extra payment for it. Over half of the consultants with management responsibilities (52%) said that they spent less than 5 hours a week on management activities, 32% spent from 5 to 10 hours a week and 13% spent over 10 hours. These figures corresponded closely to the pattern among the UK doctors.

Management training received

Among the Irish consultants who responded, only 28% had attended a management course in the past five years. The figure for the UK was 45%. Many Irish consultants reported having received such training while working abroad, in either the UK or the USA. The main providers of such training in Ireland were the Royal College of Surgeons and the IPA. Irish senior registrars had received more management training than Irish consultants had – 44% of them had attended a management course. They also tended to have attended longer courses, most commonly the Diploma in Management for Medical Doctors, provided by the Royal College of Surgeons and the IPA.

Irish consultants who had received management training tended to be less satisfied than either their UK counterparts or the senior registrars.

The need for future management training

Interestingly, Irish consultants surveyed were most likely to see a personal need for management training in the future – 77% as compared to 73% in the UK or 56% of Irish senior registrars. The kind of course that was rated most highly by both Irish consultants and senior registrars was one that aimed 'to improve techniques of strategic management e.g. strategy, service planning, forecasting, etc.'.

Respondents were asked to rate a number of management topics in terms of how useful they would find training in the topic concerned. The results are given in Table 14.1.

It can be seen from Table 14.1 that the top five choices of Irish consultants in order of priority were service planning, strategic planning, information systems, motivating staff and time management. Senior registrars chose motivating staff, selecting staff, information systems, strategic planning and the legal responsibilities of doctors. The two groups were in absolute agreement on the least relevant topics. These were equal opportunities, the work of healthcare managers, issues of health and social gain, determining the health needs of an area/community, and group behaviour. This pattern of preferences was broadly similar to that of the UK sample.

Format of training

A frequent problem with the provision of management training for doctors is to find a way of fitting it into their work schedule. The majority of consultants and senior registrars expressed a preference for training to be provided outside normal working hours, on either weekday evenings or Saturdays. If a course were longer than 8 hours most would prefer it to be split into a number of separate weekly instalments rather than run to several consecutive days. For courses longer than 40 hours, preferences were split, as indicated in Table 14.2.

About half of consultants and senior registrars would prefer to receive management training in courses that are solely for doctors. Almost a third would like to receive management training with others in the health services. About 15% would like to be trained with managers of all kinds.

Table 14.1. Rating of potential usefulness of course topics

Rank order of topics deemed most useful

Consultants (Ireland)	**Consultants (UK)**	**Senior registrars (Ireland)**
Service planning	Local budgeting	Motivating staff
Strategic planning	Business planning	Selecting staff
Information systems	Information system	Information systems
Motivating staff	Strategic planning	Strategic planning
Time management	Legal responsibilities	Legal responsibilities
Negotiating skills	Negotiating skills	Service planning
Computing skills	Motivating staff	Negotiating skills
Local budgeting	Computing skills	Reviewing staff
Service management and quality	Appraising staff	Appraising staff
Legal responsibilities of doctors	Chairing committees	Time management

Rank order of topics deemed least useful

Equal opportunities	Presentation skills	Equal opportunities
The work of healthcare managers	Equal opportunities	The work of healthcare managers
Issues of health and social gain	Health of the Nation issues	Issues of health and social gain
Determining the health needs of an area/ community	Group behaviour	Determining the health needs of an area/ community
Group behaviour	The work of NHS managers	Group behaviour

Table 14.2. Preferred timing of courses

Timing of course	Consultants	Senior registrars
One day per week	17%	3%
One half day per week	20%	25%
One evening per week	27%	28%
Two/three-day modules	20%	13%
One five-day module course	20%	41%
No response	6%	6%
	(208)	(32)

The doctors surveyed were also asked to indicate what conditions, if any, would facilitate their attendance at a management training course. The factors specified most often included:

- time off or leave to attend courses, and/or locum cover to be provided
- more information on courses available
- funding to be made available
- convenient local location (especially for doctors from outside Dublin)
- courses to be provided at convenient times.

Senior registrars indicated that time off and funding being made available would facilitate their attendance at such courses.

The consultants were also asked if they wished to make any additional comment about management training. Some of the comments were especially interesting. They suggested that management training for doctors would be of limited use unless there was a clear commitment from management that doctors be given a meaningful managerial role. Others pointed out that doctors must be given incentives to become more involved in management. From those who were already involved in, or interested in developing further their involvement in, management came the suggestion that a small group of senior medical managers should be formed and should maintain contact for purposes of communication and development. Perhaps most importantly, however, several indicated that there was a need for doctors and managers to sit down together and improve understanding of each other's roles.

Discussion

The relatively low response rate to the postal survey might lead one to suspect that the interest in assuming a greater managerial role among Irish hospital doctors is not as great as that observed by the Buckley Review Group. The response rate was certainly disappointingly low, both from consultants and senior registrars, particularly if one compares it to the response rates achieved in the UK. However, there may be a number of reasons for this, such as the sponsorship of the surveys in the UK, the longer history of clinical involvement in management in the UK, and the impact of resource management initiatives. An important factor may be the fact that no reminder letters were issued. When a comparable questionnaire was issued to UK consultants in 1987 without any reminder letter (Horsley *et al.*, 1996), however, a response rate of 48% was achieved. This compares with our response rate of 24% from consultants. If one were to take the response rate alone as an indicator of the level of interest in management and management training among Irish doctors, one would have to conclude that the level of interest is not high.

The proportion of Irish consultants who said that they had additional management responsibilities is surprisingly high compared to that in the UK. It could be that there is a significantly higher involvement by consultants in management in Ireland than is currently presumed. The examination of the types of managerial responsibilities specified indicated a wide array. Most of these related to the direct clinical responsibilities of the doctor concerned, and fewer with corporate responsibilities within a hospital outside one's own speciality area or, crucially, for managing other doctors.

Looking at the responses of senior registrars, it would seem that they are more interested in assuming a managerial role. It is also noteworthy that more of them have received management training. This suggests that future consultants will be better prepared to assume managerial roles.

As regards the content of management training for doctors, it would seem that doctors see topics such as planning, motivating staff and information systems as being priority areas. It is encouraging that so many consultants saw a need for management training for themselves in the future. How can such training be most effectively provided?

In the Irish system, in talking about management training needs, it is probably preferable to identify two levels of involvement of doctors in the management process. The first level would correspond broadly to levels 1 and 2 identified by Allen (1995). It would therefore refer to all doctors who had responsibility for managing their own practice and also had some limited involvement in hospital and departmental committees. The second level (Allen's levels 3 and 4) would include those doctors who are likely to assume a more significant managerial role as envisaged by the Buckley Review Body (Review Body on Higher Remuneration in the Public Sector, 1996). In other words, they would have to lead a distinct clinical unit with a grouping of clinical functions and would receive a payment for undertaking that work. It would also include those who currently have significant managerial and leadership responsibilities, such as Masters, RMSs and chairpersons of medical boards. The key distinction, however, would be that they would have managerial responsibility for their consultant colleagues.

The remainder of this chapter identifies some general principles which, it is suggested, should guide management training for doctors in the future.

Recommendations

Doctors should be exposed to managerial concepts and the main tenets of managerial culture at as early a stage as possible in their careers. Thus, *managerial topics should be included in the undergraduate curricula of medical schools.*

While all doctors manage, they do not all see themselves as managing nor are they all interested in management training. This suggests that, *initially at least, resources should be invested in addressing the management training needs of those doctors who express an interest.*

The depth and range of management training programmes for doctors should vary depending on the degree of managerial responsibility to be assumed by the doctor concerned. All doctors have some managerial responsibility and hence all would benefit from some understanding of basic managerial concepts and skills (although not all might want it). *There is a need for a basic management development programme for doctors that would serve as a foundation programme.* This would improve their practice of management and increase understanding across the two cultures – the managerial and the medical. (At the same time, it must be recognised that managers also need to acquire some understanding of the medical culture, and it is noteworthy that the Royal College of Surgeons has recently run some seminars on medical issues for managers.)

Doctors themselves, as indicated by our survey results, have indicated a preference for receiving management training in the company of other doctors. *All basic management development programmes for doctors should therefore be provided on a unidisciplinary basis.* All doctors need some basic managerial awareness in order to operate effectively within their working environment. This basic managerial knowledge and skill can be delivered in the form of formal training courses which could be adapted to fit in with the working schedule of doctors. *It is desirable that such courses be confined to doctors with the same levels of respon-*

sibility, i.e. consultants with other consultants, senior registrars with other senior registrars, etc. Apart from that, such courses need not necessarily be provided on site but could be availed of from some central location, or indeed by distance learning. If they were provided by distance learning it would be advisable to supplement them with some discussion or tutorial sessions to reinforce the learning. At all events, *the scheduling and format of all management development programmes for doctors should attempt to fit in, in an imaginative and flexible way, with the work schedule of doctors.*

It is vital that management programmes for doctors build on the existing interests, concerns and commitments of doctors themselves. Thus, for example, doctors tend to be used to more didactic forms of teaching and these should be used initially until trust is built up between the doctors and those providing the training. Also, as the results of the survey indicate, doctors are currently concerned about service planning and it could serve as a useful entry into management topics.

A distinction must be drawn between the management training needs of doctors operating at levels 1 and 2 of managerial responsibility and of those operating at levels 3 and 4. *The difficulties and the challenges for doctors assuming enhanced managerial roles, particularly where these involve managing other doctors, must not be underestimated. Special initiatives are needed to support them.* They will need the following.

1. *Advanced management development programmes for doctors*, as a priority. If a cadre of doctors within a hospital were to be assuming new management responsibilities, it would be desirable that they be developed together, on site. The content of the programme could then be tailored to address their particular and enhanced needs. There would be the added benefit of contributing to enhance communication and networking within the hospital between doctors with a managerial role.

2. *Multidisciplinary management and organisational development initiatives for themselves and their clinical and managerial colleagues to clarify roles and structures.* The point was made in the survey responses that doctors and managers need to sit down together and work out their respective roles. This is obviously a first priority and may require some outside facilitation and support. A number of workshops may be required on site to allow key players address the issues. This would take the form of both management and organisational development, and would probably include some

form of team-building. The development of service plans could provide a useful task-based focus for this work.

3. *Ongoing support from doctors engaged in similar roles from across the system.* Several of the healthcare management training schools in the UK offer facilitated learning sets for clinical and medical directors. These meet for a day at regular (monthly or bimonthly) intervals with an independent facilitator. They can provide a confidential forum in which doctors from across the country with similar responsibilities and issues can share their experiences and concerns and plan action for the future. They can therefore provide the necessary source of advice and support to doctors who are breaking new ground and trying to create new roles for themselves.

Some further principles should govern this higher-level management development, as follows.

- *The programmes should be linked as closely as possible to the working environment of the doctors concerned* (Boufford, 1994). This is to ensure their relevance, ease of transfer of learning back into the work situation, and that they fit in with the work schedule of doctors.
- Such programmes should emerge from an analysis of the local situation. *All those with a key stake in the content and outcomes of management development programmes for doctors should have input into their design and format* (Boufford, 1994). This would include doctors themselves, managers, other health professionals and patient representatives. In fact, the process of designing programmes and identifying the needs can itself be a potent force for change and development.

Efforts to provide meaningful, effective and relevant management development programmes for doctors are at the cutting edge of the clash between the medical and the managerial cultures. The way ahead must be to recognise openly that it is difficult for both cultures to change and adapt. The Irish health system differs in many respects from that of the USA and the UK in which many Irish doctors have been trained. Ways of involving doctors effectively in management in Ireland will have to be developed by building on the uniqueness of the Irish system while also learning the lessons from elsewhere.

Management development programmes for doctors should provide a safe environment in which new skills and concepts can be learned and new ways of behaving tried out. They will need to be linked with multidisciplinary organisation development initiatives.

Acknowledgements

The generous assistance of Stephen Horsley, Emilie Roberts, Diane Barwick, Steve Barrow and David Allen in making their questionnaire available to me for use in this study is gratefully acknowledged.

CHAPTER 15

Leadership: Making the Best Use of the Nursing Resource

GERALDINE MCCARTHY

Introduction

The late 1980s and early 1990s saw the publication of a number of reports on the future of the Irish health services, with particular emphasis on reforms involving a managerial role for staff directly concerned. These include the Commission on Health Funding (1989), the Dublin Hospital Initiative Group Reports (Kennedy Reports) (1990, 1991), The Efficiency Review of Acute Hospitals (Fox Report) (Department of Health, 1990, 1991), the Advisory Expert Committee on Local Government Reorganisation and Reform (Barrington Report) (Department of the Environment, 1987), *Shaping a Healthier Future* (Department of Health, 1994) and a document on the education and training of nurses (An Bord Altranais, 1994). It is acknowledged that healthcare reforms will bring challenges and opportunities to strengthen the services through more effective management, increase the managerial role of doctors and nurses, heighten concern to use existing resources more effectively, and emphasise quality control. This has implications for resource management in nursing and for the leadership necessary to respond to the challenges presented.

This chapter briefly describes leadership and its relationship to nursing and resource management. It proposes that leadership in Irish nursing requires strengthening, and that transformational leadership is needed in a changing healthcare system which requires professional managers who are knowledgeable, skilful and competent. Jaques' (1990) Stratified System Theory (SST) is explained and applied to resource management. The chapter also describes the work necessary with respect to resource management at executive, middle and first-line nurse management levels.

Leadership and nursing

Definitions of leadership abound. It has been considered a dynamic, group process whereby one individual influences all other group members to achieve objectives (Bernard and Walsh, 1995); a process of influencing the activities of a group towards goal setting and achievements (Stogdill, 1986); a social transaction (Merton, 1969); and a process of persuasion and example by which an individual induces group action in accord with the leader's purpose (Gardner, 1986). Lundborg (1982) states that a leader can transform a crowd into a well functioning organisation. Leaders set and shape the culture in organisations (Rafferty, 1993) and develop organisational capacity (Cole, 1993). Embodied in all definitions are the concepts of leader, follower, group, process and goals. Over the years, nurse leaders have emerged, with well-known figures such as Nightingale and Henderson receiving international acclaim. Each country has its nurse leaders and these are a product of education, experience and mentoring.

Types of leadership are charismatic, traditional, situational, functional, transactional and transformational. An early theory of leadership is trait, which infers that leaders have many personality, intellectual and ability traits and that leadership can be learned (Bernard & Walsh, 1995). Situational theory explores leadership context in particular situations at a particular point in time. Inter-actional theory is a combination of trait and situational theory, and proposes that what matters is the interaction between the leader and followers in specific problem situations.

Transformational leadership is perceived as essential for today's organisation (Bernard & Walsh, 1995) and is defined as commitment and empowering followers to achieve a vision (Burns, 1978) even if the need for change is not appreciated. Transforming leaders are inno-vative and evolutionary and develop role-independence (Gardner, 1986). It is a style of leadership that focuses on a commitment to change, ability to re-conceptualise systems and build networks, relationships, tolerance for complexity and production of creative work. The transformational leader is capable of making strategic decisions alone but after deliberations with others; is committed to the organisation; and has long-term and dynamic vision of what can be accomplished (Burns, 1978). Requirements for transformational leadership are the power to deal with complexity, ambiguity and uncertainty, and the ability to empower and inspire others through communication of a vision of what is to be accomplished (Daft, 1992). Wolf (1986), in studying nurse leaders, says that transformational leaders communicate trust through decentralisation and participation. However, in Irish nursing to date very few transforming leaders have emerged.

In contrast, transactional leadership is oriented towards completing the task at hand and maintaining the *status quo*. The person who operates in a transactional manner, according to Burns (1978), is in a caretaking role, has no vision of what could be and conveys little inspiration to others. Instead this leader makes a trade-off with followers to meet explicit or implicit goals. Transactional leadership has operated almost exclusively, and has been very strong at all levels of management, in Irish nursing. While serving the health service well in the production of efficient and quick responses, it has existed to the detriment of image and the evolution of the role of nurses in health service management.

Leadership style is related to the amount of control or freedom afforded followers, and three recognised styles exist: autocratic, democratic, *laissez-faire*. Research has shown that those subjected to autocratic leadership became progressively more submissive; those subjected to democratic leadership became more cohesive; those subjected to *laissez-faire* leadership became less productive and satisfied (Stogdill, 1986). With respect to nursing, autocratic style has been used most often, with resultant stifling of initiative.

Few studies (Rafferty, 1993; McCloskey & Molen, 1987) exist on leadership in nursing. Rafferty (1993) proposes that nurses have been socialised into deferential roles. Her research, which involved interviews with 30 UK nurses in leadership positions, showed that they believed leadership qualities emerged early and included enthusiasm, liveliness, vision, communication ability, persuasiveness and nonjudgemental skills. Further, it was suggested that leadership can be learned, preferably through role models and mentors. Overall, two major themes emerged from the research: leadership as a constellation of qualities and attributes, and leadership as a process of influencing and managing change. The respondents in the study also stated that leaders in nursing 'rescue nursing from being an invisible but necessary service'. Rafferty (1993) questions nursing's ability to promote a leadership culture and consciousness. One must query the influence gender exerts in this phenomenon.

Lack of leadership is particularly evident at policy level, where there is inadequate consultation and articulation of what is best from a nursing perspective. For example, there is a dearth of nurse member-ship on policy-framing committees, and a lack of documents produced by nurse leaders on specific issues, i.e. those relating to the strategic direction or changes in health service provision, or to changes in nurse education. Similarly, there is a dearth of nursing representation on the media when relevant issues are being discussed and represented at senior management levels or on political bodies. From experience, the author suggests that Irish nurse leaders in the main have been the products of autocratic systems and mentored into using primarily transactional styles. Leaders of the past have shaped a culture which socialised nurses into deferential roles. However, a few nurse leader/managers have worked to empower others to rescue nursing from being an invisible but necessary service. While training for manage-ment has been provided for many nurses, either it was not the appropriate type of training to produce leaders or else it is not possible to learn leadership if cognitive ability is insufficient.

Management of the human resource

Management is the process of getting the work done by other people, and of leading those managed towards organisational goals. Human resource management is defined as all management decisions and actions that affect the nature of the relationship between organisation and employees (Gunnigle & Flood, 1990). It aims to ensure quality services through matching resources to need. It is increasingly impor-tant (Cowling & Mailer, 1990) under circumstances where patient throughput, complexity of care and consumer awareness increase and while resources are finite, thereby forcing individuals to work harder to meet demands.

Leadership is evident when the appointed head, due to situation and positional authority, leads the group members to accept directives without any apparent exertion of force (Holloman, 1985). In the literature the concepts of manager and leader are intrinsically inter-linked. It may be said that nursing is over-managed but under-led. At this time of great change in the health service, nurse managers are involved primarily at three levels in resource management: executive (chief nurse), middle (unit/divisional) and first line. The respon-sibilities of each of these will be addressed later in this chapter as they pertain to hospital nurse management.

Jaques' organisational theory: management and leadership

Jaques, a psychoanalyst and management consultant, proposes an organisational theory developed over 40 years and published in 16 texts (see Jaques, 1990; Jaques & Clement, 1991). It has been claimed that companies which used the theory reported almost mystical results, including leaps in productivity and happier, more dedicated employees (Ross, 1992). The author, having worked with the theory in an organisation employing 900 nurses, believes it offers a framework of insights that explains organisational behaviour which is useful in resource management. Jaques (1990) proposes that natural hierarchies assert themselves whenever humans organise themselves to work. The hierarchies relate to levels of work and levels of human capacity. The levels of work depend on the complexity of work to be done within the organisation and the trick in management, Jaques (1990) suggests, is to match the worker to the work (see Fig. 15.1).

Jaques' Stratified Systems Theory (SST) proposes that individuals' problem-solving abilities develop through youth and maturity in predictable patterns. He asserts that individuals have an inherent potential for cognitive development and are accordingly equipped to rise only so high and no higher in any organisation. Further, he says that no amount of positive thinking or education can change the potential to approach problems in increasingly complex ways. Jaques states that some people are born with the ability to become leaders at CEO level, some at middle management level, and some people are not, and never will be, managerial material but are more focused on the here and now and happy to work operationally under the direction of a manager who will guide the work. There are natural work hierarchies and there are people who are naturally endowed to occupy roles within the different levels (Jaques, 1990).

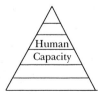 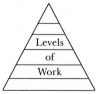

Fig. 15.1. Levels of work and capacity

Jaques warns that it takes 5–10 years for a top manager to turn around an organisation and the systems working within it, so that it enhances human effectiveness and creativity and allows individuals to reach their potential. He also states that companies get into trouble when the layers on their organisational charts fail to correspond to the structures needed, and when managers are not clearly accountable for managerial work. In testing principles which differentiate one level of work from another, Jaques proposes this has to do with the target completion time of the longest task or project assigned to that role. Some people, according to Jaques (1990), cannot see past their next pay cheque and usually end up in low-level work. A few are endowed with the gift to foresee across decades. In between are the rest of the workforce; the level of sophistication with which individuals approach problems determines where in the cognitive hierarchy they belong. Jaques (1990) has identified various levels of cognitive ability, ranging from the very concrete ('tell me what to do') to the very abstract, in which a person is capable of imagining several chains of possible consequences and related outcome. When a manager's cognitive abilities fail to match the hierarchy level occupied, the company shrinks down to the manager's level; but when hierarchies correspond to capacity, the organisation thrives. Leadership, for Jaques (1990), depends on cognitive capacity and work comparable to this capacity.

Application of SST to nurse management

A number of important propositions outlined above have relevance to nurse management. Resource management entails setting up clearly differentiated roles with explicit levels of authority and accountability. It involves recruiting appropriate people to perform the necessary work (Cowling and Mailer, 1990). Jaques (1990) explains that both work and human capacity are arranged in a hierarchy and that capacity determines the ability to deal with work complexity. This has implications for identification of work and human capacity, for recruitment practices and for delegation of accountability. He also discusses how managers can delegate accountability for work completion while still allowing subordinates to develop and follow the path created by themselves. Hospitals where the majority of nurses work are called hybrid organisations (Jaques, 1990): that is, there are some employees who function within a hierarchical structure while working alongside autonomous professionals in the same organisation. This represents nursing and medicine (the two greatest resources) as they operate at present within hospital structures. Nurse management in hospitals will be used for the remainder of this chapter to discuss resource management.

When SST is applied it means that very few nurses may have the ability to work at executive level where work complexity is greatest and where transformational abilities and skills are necessary. It also means that many nurses content to work at lower levels should not be encouraged to progress up the work hierarchy. What has happened over the years is that many clinical nurses who were job-satisfied in mostly transactional patient–nurse relationships were promoted to ward sister or chief nurse positions which proved both non-satisfying and beyond individual capability. The author contends that this trend needs reversal, as it is to the detriment of clinical nursing and nurse management. What is necessary is to identify potential, mentor and develop it to its full capacity.

Jaques (1990) maintains that progressive management requires a decentralised system of decision-making and accountability held at the appropriate level. *Shaping a Healthier Future* (Department of Health, 1994), the Audit Commission (1992) and the current nursing literature state that organisational structures within nursing are functioning inadequately, with poor authority and accountability specification. There is also a recognised need, as seen in recent unrest in the nursing profession, to redefine roles and associated account-ability. Thus, the traditional levels of management which have existed in nursing over the years need to be examined in terms of requirement and role, and it appears that this might be done by the recently established Commission on Nursing. The work to be done at each level of management needs to be differentiated in terms of explicit outputs to be achieved (Dublin Hospital Initiative Group, 1990; Jaques, 1990). Also, a decentralised system of accountability and decision-making needs to be established. Based on the literature reviewed and on experience, the author proposes that the following simple organisational structure should exist:

- *Director of Nursing*
- *Divisional Nurse Managers*
- *First-Line Managers.*

It is suggested that this should consist of one nurse manager at executive level, a number of divisional managers who manage resources across wards/units/community care areas, and first-line operational managers. To date, other nurse managers have filled a single responsibility role across services such as staff scheduling or quality assurance. These roles should be removed from the organisation, and the work done incorporated into the role responsibilities of the three levels of managers listed above.

Those three levels of managers should operate autonomously through interlinked strategy and policies, and carry 24-hour responsibility. Each higher level should be responsible (at different levels) for a number of functions such as those shown as appropriate for hospital managers in Fig. 15.2. These relate to resource management, and emerged from focus group research carried out as part of a research and development project (McCarthy, 1993a, 1993b).

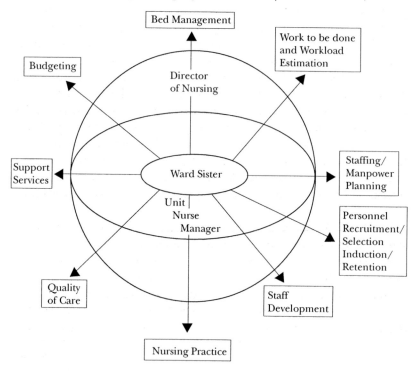

Fig. 15.2. Areas of accountability within a requisite nursing management structure

The structure should be overt and explicit. Work at director level should be strategic; at divisional level it should comprise planning and implementation of policies; and work at first line should be operational. Work level, required abilities, predominant leadership style and skills are listed in Table 15.1.

For the remainder of the chapter the work of each of the three levels of management is discussed in relation to present arrangements and future trends. Overall, the ideas expressed are based on the experience of the research and development project referred to above.

Director of Nursing

Present arrangements

The necessity for a Director of Nursing arises out of the proportion of nurses within any healthcare organisation, the need to manage proactively and lead this resource, and the overall effects of nursing numbers on budget, quality of care, technological advances, etc. (Jaco *et al.*, 1994). In the Irish healthcare system these managers have been entitled Directors of Nursing, Matrons or Chief Nursing Officers and have been recruited through the Local Appointments Commission. Nurse managers at this level are supported by a deputy (sometimes) and by varying numbers of assistant matrons or nursing officers. No nurse in the country is occupying a higher level managerial position.

Transactional leadership has typically been displayed where the nurse manager is a general manager of day-to-day nursing operations. Planning staffing levels and functions, creating an effective organisational structure and directing nursing work, even at the lowest

Table 15.1. Work level, predominant leadership style, and skills required for different levels of nurse manager

Level	Work	Ability	Leadership style	Skill
Director	Strategic	Complex & cognitive	Transformational +++ Transactional +	Creative Visitionary
Divisional	Operational	Complex & concrete	Transformational + Transactional +	Identifying Planning Establishing systems
First line	Operational	Concrete	Transactional	Operational

level, are chief functions. Networks of co-operative relationships have evolved, medical consultants frequently discuss staffing or related issues, and problems are solved in a transactional manner. As a result of difficult cases, methods (e.g. the discharge of a particular patient) or functions of individuals (e.g. nurses) change but the process does not alter inherently and the change is not sustained. There has been a lack of strategic planning and of the knowledge and information which underlies this activity.

The system has endured through recruitment practices; poor remuneration; mentoring by older and more experienced matrons who have trained in the same system; lack of basic 'back-up' resources including divisional nurse managers who would constantly take responsibility for divisions, secretarial support and education for higher level work. Responsibilities in policy-making, planning and programme direction in the assurance of quality are not normally included as part of the role.

Gunnigle & Flood (1990) assert that first-class managers are also first-class leaders and distinguish themselves in thinking long-term, looking beyond the unit managed, reaching and influencing individuals beyond boundaries; emphasising vision, political skills, and revision of essential processes. This would correlate with the vision of Jaques (1990) in terms of how the most senior manager should operate in a transformational manner. However, to date there has been little time or support for Directors to develop as outlined above. As a result they have been inhibited from contributing in a more meaningful way to economic debate, from interpreting nursing to Boards of Directors, CEOs and consumers; and in bargaining for available resources (Davidson, 1990; Jaco *et al.*, 1994).

Future trends

A major function of the Director of Nursing is to create and maintain a culture within which professional nursing can be practised and to provide leadership which facilitates and encourages involvement of staff in decision-making processes (Deal & Kennedy, 1982). A good environment does not just happen – leadership is necessary to bring it about. Experienced directors know that a culture exists and realise the enormous impact the general mood, tenor, or character has on the overall success and quality of services. Directors have worked over the years to maintain a culture, but some non-nurse managers lack an understanding of its worth, perhaps because the culture was not always appropriate for advancement.

Some writers propose that, in creating new structures, there is no need for a nurse at executive level (Rafferty, 1993; Rice, 1987). The author contends that without a nurse at executive level there would be no organisational nursing culture across services, no one nurse would know and hold responsibility for nursing, and the organisation would be ineffective from a nursing perspective. However, the director must be progressive and credible, must mobilise commitment and must understand how all parts of the organisation interact and are affected by internal or external changes.

Task force documents to aid Directors of Nursing in the organisation of nursing services and associated managerial accounability have been developed in the USA by the Joint Commission on Accreditation of Hospitals (Mayer *et al.*, 1990), and in the UK (Lathlean, 1988). These documents offer guidance on creating an environment for reform; deciding nursing service priorities and articulating them through a written nursing philosophy; redesigning nursing management and nursing care delivery systems to make optimal use of nursing resources; collection and analysis of information; and promoting interdisciplinary collaboration between nursing, medicine and administration. They also identify elements for which strategic plans and policies should be articulated. In the absence of national criteria for Irish nurse managers, but perhaps using those produced by the Irish Matrons' Association (1995), it is suggested that leaders in director positions include in their strategic plans the elements outlined in Fig. 15.2.

An appraisal of Irish nurse management suggests that strategic direction for nursing at the highest level is poorly developed and that the leadership required at present may be inadequate. The question then arises: who can do this for Irish nursing? Rice (1987) questions whether nursing is able to produce individuals to fill key positions at strategic level, which requires a different type of thinking than that used at operational level. He agrees with Jaques (1990) that such an individual needs high conceptual ability and capability. Rafferty (1993) questions nursing's ability to promote a leadership culture and consciousness. What appears to be needed is the recruitment of individuals with potential, the provision of education and some mentoring by appropriate personnel. Work was done in a major hospital in Dublin in which the present author worked as Research and Development Manager, and included statements on all the elements in Fig. 15.2. Strategic direction was set by the director, new job descriptions outlining accountability and outputs were developed for unit and first-line managers, and innovative arrangements were made and tested.

Management at divisional level

Present arrangements

Some services have clearly established divisions of operation based on medical case mix and/or intensity of work. Within these, nurse managers are called assistant directors of nursing, unit/divisional managers and assistant chief nursing officers. However, methods of recruitment and job descriptions vary considerably. Some of the managers have developed a work role in just one area, e.g. bed management or staff scheduling. There is also considerable general shared responsibility due to work rota systems, and considerable 'acting up' for the director or 'acting down' for first-line managers when deemed necessary. The role is more administrative than managerial, and leads to confusion for staff with respect to whom to approach to discuss, for example, working arrangements, career plans, educational or skill training requirements. Staff very often bypass this level of administrator and discuss matters with the director.

Future trends

From a resource perspective, nurse managers functioning at this level should ensure effective and efficient use of limited resources, agree ways of operating services (Rice, 1987) and collaborate with medical colleagues in decision-making about all facets of the service (Costain, 1990). Key management functions should operate under the policy guidelines set by the Director of Nursing. Activities could include, for example (see Fig. 15.2), supervision and development of first-line managers; monitoring and controlling the work flowing into the unit through bed management in agreement with consultant colleagues, or operated in relation to service plans; planning, costing, implementing and evaluating developments in services; establishing and implementing systems to evaluate workload and plan staffing; recruiting of staff and maintenance of personnel data and the nursing

establishment; ensuring the operation of induction and staff development programmes; applying systems for evaluating nursing practice
and quality of care; establishing, monitoring and negotiating support
services; and detailed control of the nursing budget. The work may
also mean redefining work, adding new services and roles. This
description is similar to that outlined as being appropriate by the
Joint Commission on Accreditation of Hospitals (Kramer, 1990), but
is rarely seen in Irish nursing. The manager should hold 24-hour
accountability for the service and mentor competent first-line
managers to 'act up' when appropriate during the 24-hour, seven-day
week for which the nursing resource must be managed.

As skill-mix initiatives and models of care delivery are central to
the work of this manager, they are now described in some detail.

Skill mix and staffing

Very few Irish nurse managers have enough available data on which
to base decisions and argue challenges regarding staff utilisation. This
in part has been due to the lack of computer technology which makes
the data more easily available. Barton (1993, p. 16) wrote that 'the
policy decision by the Department to relate hospital budgets to outputs
has created a new climate in which providers of healthcare must define
and justify the services they provide'. For nurse managers at division
level, there is therefore a real danger that a diagnostic related groups
(DRG) case mix will be used for funding services which will allow
similar resources for DRGs with similar treatment processes without
integration of nursing management data. A responsibility of the
divisional nurse manager, in this author's opinion, is adequate costing
of the nursing resource, and this cannot be done without detailed
nursing workload and establishment data and utilisation of computerised databases including a nursing minimum data set (Sermeus
& Delesie, 1992).

Most of the patient classification systems in common use to
identify the work to be done for patients were not designed for the
type of patient now using the health services, such as the medically
complex, aged, and day care. Patient dependency classification systems
are important in estimating workload, but they need to be integrated
with information on admitting diagnoses, problems requiring nursing
interventions, length of stay and quality measures to build realistic
profiles (Van Hoesen & Eriksen, 1990). Correlations with DRGs are

possible with the use of nursing diagnosis or of national endeavours such as those developed in Belgium, where a nursing minimum data set is collected in all hospitals four times a year during a 15-day sampling period and used for funding (Sermeus & Delesie, 1992), or across European countries (Mortensen, 1994), or through the International Council of Nurses' work to relate nursing diagnosis to DRGs (Fitzpatrick *et al.*, 1989) and to describe the contribution of nurses to care. All this information should be known and used by nurse managers in resource management at unit level.

In the hospital research and development project referred to above, data on bed utilisation, medical diagnosis and patient dependency on nursing care were produced for each ward and collated for each division. It was then possible to make comparisons across wards and divisions. Some work was also commenced in relation to matching DRG with nursing diagnosis, in an effort to differentiate patient dependency on nursing care for patients with similar medical diagnoses. This information aided decisions on resource utilisation.

Models of care delivery: nurses, support workers and skill mix

In an effort to match the work to the worker, the responsibility of divisional nurse managers should include, in collaboration with first-line managers, the recruitment of staff. While this responsibility has been devolved in a few agencies in the Irish healthcare service, in many more it is a centralised function whereby staff are selected for positions without full recognition of the work they are expected to do or the team they are expected to join. Divisional managers should know the work profile of each nurse employee and recognise it in terms of the work she or he is capable of doing as a team member when placed with others in a particular ward/division. Recognition of skill competency level on a continuum from novice to expert in a particular clinical area, as suggested by Benner and Wrubel (1993), is vital. The possession of such data helps in building up stable teams of competent experienced nurses to give quality care.

A resource problem for many hospitals is the employment of too many junior newly qualified nurses who have inadequate skills or knowledge for effective working without close supervision. The author suggests that what may be wrong is staff nurse mix rather than volume of nurses, and without knowledge of expertise levels this will continue to be the case. In the R&D project the methods described above were operationalised, and recruitment responsibilities were devolved with good effect.

The question of work appropriate to nurses and other health carers will continue to be a resource management issue, and may grow in importance as Irish student nurses are removed from the workforce as a result of the changes currently being implemented in the training and education of student nurses (An Bord Altranais, 1994). Despite numerous efforts to quantify patients' acuity or nurse and 'nurse assistant' workload, and to capture the appropriate fit between level of work complexity and ability of the worker (Edwardson & Giovannetti, 1992; Ball *et al.*, 1989; Treacy, 1988), studies are generally disappointing. The author suggests that the results may be no match for discretionary, knowledgeable professional judgement at the lowest level possible in relation to level of work, individual capacity and human resource utilisation (Jaques, 1990).

Many healthcare agencies throughout the world have developed models of care delivery using other care workers to aid the nurse in delivering care (Garfink *et al.*, 1991; Workman, 1996). However, other hospitals and healthcare organisations, in managing the nursing resource and working on research findings such as those by Chang (1995), have decided to return to an almost all-nursing workforce and have introduced primary or case management systems of nursing (Kramer, 1990) to manage effectively the resource available – e.g. the ProACT model in New Jersey (Rossi *et al.*, 1990). There are some valuable lessons to be learned from the literature in relation to the mistakes that have been made in skill mix to the detriment of quality. While some costs decreased in hospitals where other team members were introduced to deliver patient care, the quality of care suffered (Buchan & Ball, 1991) and hospitals were forced to employ quality control managers.

Employment of large numbers of care assistants in the Irish healthcare system, if necessary, will require strategic planning and clarification of roles and responsibilities. Knowledge and effective leadership on the part of the director and divisional manager and a system of devolved decision-making should ensure that responsibility for skill mix and staffing and the resultant budget is placed at as low a level as possible. Accountability for induction, deciding the work appropriate to the role of each worker and appraisal of work must also be placed at this level.

Finally, for resource management at division level, information should also be available on rostered utilisation of resources as detailing in the number of nursing hours (Reid, 1987) available to patients each day and night (NHPPD and NHPPN) for each unit in terms of medical diagnosis or nursing patient dependency classification. Shift overlaps should be reduced to a minimum, as the Audit Commission (1991) stated that shift patterns theoretically have the potential to release resources of £50 million in the UK healthcare system. Centralised staffing offices are obsolete (Kramer, 1990), and all staffing and scheduling should be decentralised to the lowest possible level.

In the research and development project, staff profiles were available to divisional managers through a computerised database, staff were recruited to fit particular vacant positions, and rosters were analysed based on NHPPD/N and examined for possible deployment of staff which was then implemented at ward/unit level. Shift overlaps were reduced and, after examination of specific job specifications, new roles were described, implemented and monitored.

First-line management

Present arrangements

In the author's opinion, the first-line manager is the key to human resource management and the provision of a quality and financially tight service. Managing the nursing resource in many wards means managing at least 35 workers and a pay budget of at least £600,000 per annum. The traditional Ward Sister was promoted to the position because of expertise in clinical practice and lack of other promotional opportunities.

The author believes that a good clinician is not always a good manager. The role change from provider of care to manager is a difficult transition for many nurses, who can be caught between the expectations of patients, care-givers and managers. However, bi-directional accountability is required to ensure safe and effective care of patients, assignment of work and implementation of policies. The bi-culturism causes the first-line manager to move uneasily between labour and management. The manager often reacts to situations by 'acting down', indicating either that resources are inadequate or that staff are inadequately educated to deal with situations. Leadership in the main is transactional by adjusting, adapting and facilitating adherence to functional operating systems (patient care, equipment and staffing). Overall, the role is complex, extends over 24 hours, seven days per week, and is not easily understood (Duffield, 1991); occupants are poorly paid and those recruited in the past may not have the leadership skills or ability required today.

Decentralisation and the introduction of primary nursing are two very significant and universal factors which have altered the role. The work required now and for which primarily transactional leadership is necessary involves maintaining a broad perspective on the work to be done, monitoring and intervening on a wide range of issues, uniting disparate individuals to coalesce into a tightly knit supportive team in a stimulating environment, evaluation of services, and controlling some elements of the pay and non-pay budget.

Ability to manage resources at this level encompasses the capacity to manage patient care and the allocation of resources to patients. Assignment decisions in general are based on patient needs and staff capability, and the optimum use of nursing resources has generated considerable debate in the nursing literature. The three main approaches are task allocation, team nursing and primary nursing. Each needs to be evaluated as to its potential in specific circumstances.

Future trends

The question of first-line managers in Irish nursing needs urgent examination. While role enhancement and devolution of personnel and financial responsibilities to first-line managers have occurred in other countries (Audit Commission, 1991), in Ireland a number of issues are preventing implementation. These relate to recruitment, tenure of employment, poor pay, centralised administrative functions, the employment of separate management systems for night nursing staff, knowledge and individual ability levels, a lack of leadership and a fear from other managers of role erosion. The first-line manager of the future needs to be carefully recruited for individual capability, skills and leadership ability. Their work needs to be carefully described within the director's strategic direction. It may include at ward level all or some of the elements shown in Fig. 15.2. Work outputs must be agreed with the divisional manager, who must mentor, endorse and support.

Conclusion

Leadership is a complex concept, and nursing has only begun to develop a leadership culture. This chapter suggests that leadership in Irish nursing requires strengthening, and states that in a changing healthcare system nurse management roles need revision at strategic, divisional and first-line management levels. It may be that this examination and resultant changes will be implemented as a result of the recently established Commission on Nursing.

Jaques' (1990) Stratified System Theory is discussed, and its application to nurse management and leadership described. The work currently undertaken at executive, middle and first-line nurse management is described, and some possible future trends within a hospital framework discussed. It is suggested that when nurse managers are being recruited, attention needs to be paid to matching cognitive ability to required level of work. It is also suggested that the work of the director is strategic and work at division and first-line level is operational, and that outputs may need to be set for occupants of each of these roles. As the role of the nurse manager evolves with expanding responsibilities, educational need assessment and training in leadership as well as training to maintain competencies are necessary. Finally, it is suggested that unless accountability is devolved and nurses are involved in management at all levels, the proposals in the Health Strategy will not be realised.

PART SEVEN

The Recipients of Healthcare

CHAPTER 16

Community Participation in Primary Healthcare

JOHN KEVANY

> Community participation is, at worst, rhetoric used to gain prestige, recognition and financial support. At best, it has the greatest potential of all to bring the best health improvements to the world's poorest people. (Rifkin, 1985)

The background

This chapter explores the concepts, applications and issues of community participation in primary healthcare in Ireland. As this type of participation is relatively new to much of the developed world, it is appropriate to examine the philosophy and assumptions that underlie the process and to describe an implementation sequence based on experience to date.

Experience of community participation in healthcare planning is derived principally from development programmes in low-income countries. Community involvement is a central tenet of the WHO Declaration of Alma Ata on primary healthcare (WHO/UNICEF, 1978), to which the Irish Government is a signatory. This states that 'people have the right and the duty to participate both individually and collectively in the planning and implementation of their healthcare'. This statement applies particularly to the broader definition of primary healthcare which includes health promotion and disease prevention and which envisages the involvement of sub-professional workers.

Perceptions of community participation vary in relation to social context and to the expectations of the proponents. At one extreme is the formal *post hoc* consultation with community representatives to obtain support for plans developed by statutory agencies. At the other extreme is the direct and continuous involvement of the community in planning, managing and resourcing its primary care system. The former involves no sharing of power or authority and seeks only to gain approval for plans developed unilaterally, while the latter is based on a substantial transfer of control and responsibility to the community. Implicitly this transfer reduces the administrative and resource control of statutory agencies and emphasises instead their normative, co-ordinating and technical assistance functions.

Health needs are conventionally identified by standardised epidemiological methods usually classified under the heading of quantitative assessment. If community perceptions and preferences are to be central to the planning process, other forms of appraisal are needed which derive principally from sociological and anthropological research and which are often described as qualitative methods. To ensure that epidemiological and social dimensions of healthcare are addressed in an integrated manner, both types of assessment are required (Pope & Mays, 1995). In this context, *Shaping a Healthier Future*, published by the Department of Health (1994), states that 'it would assist the decision-making process if it was possible to devise some means of identifying and informing the preferences of the public in general between alternative priorities' and that strategy should 're-orientate the decision making process towards more open and explicit choice mechanisms which take account not only of detailed information and analysis but which also strive to reflect the public's preferences to whatever degree is possible'. These statements suggest, in the first place, a process of consultation rather than participation, and secondly they imply a categorical difference between quantitative and qualitative data. The term 'detailed information and analysis' indicates reliance on epidemiological methods, in contrast to 'striving to reflect the public's preferences', which implies that qualitative studies are not detailed and cannot be subject to similar analysis. In another policy document, on women's health (Department of Health, 1995a), reference is made to the importance of direct consultation with women to determine issues of most concern to them, but the scope and procedures of such consultation are not defined. In a subsequent statement on health promotion strategy (Department of Health, 1995b), there is no mention of consultation with, or direct participation by, the community in planning the proposed strategy. Project experience in Ireland (see below) indicates that communities have clear priorities for healthcare provision and have specific preferences on how these should be addressed.

The rationale

In conditions where human and financial resources for healthcare are severely limited, it is essential that these be used in the most efficient manner. To ensure both effectiveness and efficiency, services should respond as closely as possible to community perceptions of need and expectations of response. Failure to incorporate such a dimension in the planning process will result in lower efficiency, as well as limiting the commitment of community resources. Today, community participation in primary care planning is being explored in high-income economies for political, social and economic reasons. Democratisation of public-sector planning, progressive decentralisation of administrative functions, greater public interest in health issues and the inexorable rise in costs of care all demand a new approach to the way in which primary care systems are designed and operated (Hunt, 1990).

In the absence of a widely accepted definition of community participation in healthcare, the following description was developed for operational purposes: substantive and continuous involvement of the community in the design, management and resourcing of its primary care system (Quirke *et al.*, 1994). In the Irish context there are usually five or six groups involved in this process: the community itself, local health service staff, general medical practitioners, voluntary groups, managerial staff of the area health authority and, optionally, institutional sources of technical assistance. Commitment to such a process is complicated to some extent by the fact that general medical practitioners are independent providers of care and consequently their co-operation cannot necessarily be assumed.

The expected benefits to be derived from community participation include:

- improvement in the design and operation of primary care services, in response to user needs and preferences
- increased effectiveness and efficiency of delivery systems through wider uptake and more appropriate use of services
- active monitoring and evaluation of performance by the community arising from a clearer understanding of objectives, processes and outcomes
- increased commitment of resources by the community to a system over which it exercises greater control.

Implicit in the realisation of these benefits is a progressive assumption of responsibility for healthcare by the community, with active provision of technical and administrative support from the health authority. While the expectation of such benefits may appear reasonable, it is appropriate to consider the underlying assumptions and to examine their strengths and weaknesses.

Design and operation

Where the healthcare preferences of the community have been widely canvassed and subsequently prioritised, it can be assumed that their incorporation in the planning process will lead to improvement in the design and implementation of new services or in the modification of existing services. A potential weakness in this reasoning is that community preferences may be too diverse for planning purposes and may be unrealistic in terms of technical capacity and financial resources. Clearly, in the process of soliciting community opinion, it is essential to stipulate the technical and financial constraints within which services must operate. The level of community knowledge of health matters determines the degree to which preconditions or limitations of choice have to be specified; however, care should be taken that these are not used arbitrarily to protect the *status quo*. Finally, the priorities selected by the community may conflict with those derived from epidemiological assessment or with national or regional priorities, such as immunisation programmes, that have to be implemented uniformly.

Effectiveness and efficiency

Where services have been initiated or modified to meet community preferences, it can be assumed that uptake will increase as they become more user-friendly. If current services are under-utilised, increased uptake will improve efficiency in terms of lower delivery cost per beneficiary. It may also be postulated that such modifications will lead to a more logical choice of service and to greater timeliness of use. For example, if the delivery of primary medical care is modified to meet user preferences for access, it may be assumed that the inappropriate use of hospital accident and emergency services will decrease. Again, if access is improved, patients may seek care earlier in the disease process, thereby requiring simpler and lower cost treatment. If screening programmes are made more accessible, increased uptake should result in a greater number of early diagnoses, thus reducing the cost of later intervention. Similarly, if health promotion content and methods are adapted to accommodate specific attributes of the locality, it may be assumed that health behaviour change will accelerate, with earlier gains in morbidity and mortality. A potential risk at this stage is that improvements in care delivery and access arising from community-assisted design could result in temporary overload of some services.

Monitoring and evaluation

Community participation in the planning process implies an expectation that change will be implemented in a timely manner. This expectation can encourage the community to monitor change in inputs and process, as well as in longer term outcomes. It can also be involved in the selection of indicators and in the collection of underlying data, for example from service statistics and reports. Data collection, management and analysis skills are relatively widespread today, particularly in urban communities. Participatory evaluation, involving both care providers and recipients, can be organised with relatively limited skills and resources. The value of this process to the community should be self-evident as it generates transparent findings for independent interpretation.

The constraints in this process are, firstly, that the necessary voluntarism and monitoring skills may not be available in the community on a sustained basis and, secondly, that providers and their managers may be unwilling to release data and information from service sources on grounds of confidentiality. It should be noted, however, that confidentiality requirements may be used protectively by staff concerned that results may reflect adversely on their performance. Such concern is understandable, as subjectivity in the interpretation of results can lead to different conclusions being drawn by care agencies and the communities they serve.

Commitment of resources

A primary care system which has been modified to reflect community preferences and which is monitored and evaluated by the community itself represents a significant sharing of responsibility and transfer of control from providers to users. Such control encourages the community to invest its own resources in healthcare, particularly for new technologies and special services perceived to be of value. The provision of voluntary skilled time for the planning and monitoring of care is an obvious example. More extensive use of volunteer time for non-clinical services such as meals-on-wheels or home care support is another area that has been developed successfully. Fundraising for specific purposes, such as the purchase of new diagnostic or treatment equipment, is an area where substantial resources can be generated. These efforts can be further encouraged by cost-sharing with the health authority; however, such financing arrangements need to be clearly agreed before resource mobilisation is initiated. Such resource generation can also assist in containing healthcare costs by subsidising service modifications or initiating activities on a self-financing basis.

The potential risk in this area is that voluntarism may decline over time. Such attrition can be minimised if health authorities rigorously cost such voluntary activities and report them under the specific heading of community co-financing.

The process

Community participation can be developed in a range of settings and at different levels of operation. It can be applied to a geographically or administratively defined population, to a service catchment area or to demographic, ethnic or socio-economic subgroups within a specified area. In Ireland, the population of a rural district electoral division was involved over two years in the planning and development of modifications to the existing primary healthcare services, details of which are published in Quirke *et al.* (1994). A community-based primary care system is being developed for traveller families in which the families themselves participated in the baseline assessment of needs and the design of a delivery system to meet their mobile lifestyle (Eastern Health Board, 1996). A general practice in the UK initiated a community-based planning exercise to redesign the content and delivery of primary care to meet the needs of the community it served (Murray *et al.*, 1994). A WHO-sponsored 'Healthy Cities' project in Scotland strongly emphasised community involvement and control, and laid down the principles by which this could be achieved (Hunt, 1990). The development officer of an NHS locality in Newcastle organised a planning workshop on primary healthcare with a range of community interest groups (Newcastle and North Tyneside Health Authorities, 1995). These are diverse examples of community participation in primary care planning in these islands; as experience accumulates such participation will inevitably develop a more structured approach. Based on existing experience, however, key components and implementation sequences have become apparent and are presented below.

Formal commitment to participation

This may come from the community itself, from the local health authority, from independent service providers or a combination of these groups. To ensure sustainability, however, any initiative will require an institutional commitment from the local health authority to encourage and develop community capacity. These institutions are the traditional holders of bureaucratic power, and they must be prepared to share this substantially with the community if the initiative is to succeed.

Community organisation for health

This is usually initiated through existing structures to avoid alienating established interests and power bases. At this point the initiative may be taken up by such groups themselves or may be delegated to a special group that will keep them informed. This clears the way to forming a healthcare group, often composed of informed and motivated individuals who are able to devote the required time and skills to the process. Once it is formed, the terms of reference for the group can be established in consultation with the health authority and independent providers. Today many communities in Ireland have an official development group and may also have a development officer to organise their activities and generate external resources.

Preliminary identification of issues by rapid appraisal

This step determines the main issues for the healthcare agenda, so that further information-gathering can be relevant and focused. The process of obtaining reliable and representative information on community perceptions of health issues can take various forms, but it should be guided by certain principles which have been described for operational use (WHO, 1988). Anthropological research methods have been widely adapted for this purpose and include the use of key informants, focus groups and in-depth interviews, as well as the organisation of community fora where ideas can be openly debated.

Validity of information and opinion is ensured by triangulation of findings generated by different methods and sources.

Establishment of a health information base

Substantive participation of the community in healthcare requires that their representatives be involved from the outset, particularly in the planning process. This requires that they have access to comprehensive information on health status and conditions, including the provision of existing facilities and services, the cost of interventions and current budget allocations, as well as actual and potential resources. A substantial amount of this information is already available from sector and area reports, service records, case load analysis, etc. The database can be set up by the health authority, a general practice or a community development agency, depending on the resources, skills and level of interest. If the information base is not located in the community, however, it is essential that full and ready access by the community is guaranteed. For the same reason, all information compiled must be expressed or summarised in a form that is fully comprehensible to the non-specialist. While this entails additional effort by those responsible for establishing and maintaining the base, it is clearly a prerequisite for active involvement.

Community self-assessment by baseline survey

This process enables the community to generate current information on demography, epidemiology, perceived priorities, knowledge, attitudes and practices, as well as potential human and financial resources in the community. This operation is central to community involvement and control for several reasons: it enables the community to decide what information is relevant and thereby determine the agenda; it permits it to examine qualitative aspects of healthcare not usually addressed by epidemiological methods and, importantly, it gives its members experience and confidence to operate effectively in the healthcare arena. First-hand information of current conditions and a direct familiarity with personal responses obtained from doorstep interviews are of particular value in the subsequent dialogue stages described below. Self-assessment often takes the form of a household survey and requires skills in sampling, questionnaire design, data collection and analysis, as well as the ability to present results in a simplified form for non-specialised users. This process must be scientifically valid and technically reliable yet adapted to community use; university departments and specialised units of health authorities are useful sources of technical assistance at this stage. It is important that the community carries out, or at least understands, each stage of this process so that it can use the results and other outputs with confidence; experience shows that this can be achieved even where literacy barriers exist. The acquisition by members of the community of new knowledge and skills during this stage is seen as a practical benefit of voluntarism and can enhance job qualifications in areas of high unemployment.

Feedback to the community

The survey results are fed back to the community in a comprehensible manner so that the findings are widely known and understood and the democratic nature of the planning process is maintained. This operation essentially provides the community with core information to establish its internal priorities for the planning process. Results of other studies in the information base, including cost estimates, should also be made available at this stage so that the priority selection process can be fully informed. Information on unit costs of interventions and service delivery modes is essential to identifying options and establishing realistic priorities. While the health authority is the only practical source of such information it may not always be available, either because detailed costing has not been carried out or because managers are reluctant to divulge it. It is useful to assign specific areas of responsibility to individual members of the health group so that further information-gathering and case preparation can be shared and specific expertise developed. It is also important at this stage that actual and potential resources in the community are defined and that commitment to supporting specific priorities is agreed.

Dialogue workshops

These should be organised by the community to determine how its selected priorities will be addressed by care providers and by service management; these workshops should be sequential and progressive, as follows.

1. *Dialogue with care providers:* this first workshop presents the community's priorities and proposed strategy to local service providers. These include general practitioners, public health

nurses, social welfare officers, home care officers, voluntary agency staff and any other individuals providing primary care. It can include representatives from the first referral level such as the administrator or matron of the district hospital or other local health facilities. The purpose of this workshop is to expose care providers to the findings and opinions of the community and to engage in discussion on ranking, resources and feasibility. Dialogue at this level can lead to useful alliances between users and providers, based on common interests. Issues involving co-operation between users and providers can also be addressed at this level, possibly avoiding the need to carry them forward to the next stage. The findings of this workshop usually determine the agenda for the next stage.

2. *Dialogue with management:* This workshop provides the opportunity for users and providers jointly to present their priorities and suggestions to the management of the primary care system, who in turn will be responsible for assisting change and providing additional resources. Additional resources to finance change and innovation may not be as great a constraint as anticipated; some changes will improve efficiency and thereby generate savings for reallocation, while new resources in the form of community manpower and funding can reduce unforeseen demands on fixed budgets. In respect of community financing, it is useful to set up short-, medium- and long-term priorities at this stage so that fundraising targets can be set with realism and matching funds projected accordingly. It is emphasised that this workshop is not an isolated planning activity but the start of a continuing dialogue between users, providers and management on the implemen-tation of agreed changes. Priorities will be refined over time, issues will emerge and solutions evolve in an iterative fashion. Growing understanding and changing relationships between the different categories of participants emerge as they become aware of each other's agendas, strengths and constraints. The recognition of participants as individuals rather than as official representatives also produces notable improvement in the rate and quality of interaction, to the advantage of the process as a whole. Before concluding, this workshop should agree on the official status of the community group and on its continuing role in the operation of the healthcare system. Above all, this workshop should produce

266

an agreed and time-bound implementation plan that can be readily monitored by all participants.

Monitoring and evaluation

Based on an agreed implementation plan, the community health group can monitor service change against time-bound objectives. Monitoring will initially be directed at changes in inputs, procedures and outputs of the system, including changes in service uptake. Impact evaluation can be considered where rapid changes in specific morbidities or other health status indicators can be expected. Provided that the required data are routinely generated by service reports, participation in this phase by non-specialised participants is relatively straightforward. This is a sustained role for the health group and will require continuing commitment, although the amount of work involved at any time may be relatively small. Following the pattern of the planning stage, specific responsibilities can be delegated to individuals within the group so that a degree of specialised knowledge can be built up. Regular meetings of the group and service providers can review accumulated monitoring information and recommend adjustments in the implementation plan as required.

The actions of the health board to promote and support effective participation are relatively well defined. The priority assigned to the process should be reflected in all relevant policy and strategy statements and staff orientation workshops provided at all levels with particular attention to supervisors and first-line management. Specific training in the concepts, objectives and actions required for the promotion and support of participation is required for service providers, particularly those working directly with the community. In Ireland today, the public health nurse is probably best positioned technically, managerially and socially to promote this process. In practice, however, it is not a priority task and statutory functions leave little discretionary time for such work. To ensure success, protected time should be designated for this purpose and a detailed work plan developed to ensure that it is used productively. In a recent analysis of public health nursing in Ireland (National Public Health Nursing Committee, 1994), reference is made to the need for planning and coordinating primary care at the local level and to the comparative advantage of the public health nurse in involving the community in the process, yet no commitment to such a new role emerges in the conclusions.

Conclusion

A common factor in experience to date has been the need to provide technical assistance and training to the community in order that it can participate effectively. Such technical assistance can come from a variety of sources depending on local circumstances; fortunately there is a wide range of actual and potential sources of low-cost technical assistance and skills training in Ireland today. The health authority itself can provide both advisory and training support to the community, but this may be difficult to arrange within existing budgets and may introduce unwanted bias into the process. Practical and widely available sources of technical assistance are health and management departments of universities and technical colleges. Such assistance is compatible with both their teaching and research functions and provides useful material for academic projects. In addition, administrative and financial support can be obtained from local development partnerships in designated areas of disadvantage. Such support is available under a sub-programme of the Local Urban and Rural Development Programme which is administered by Area Development Management Ltd, with support from the Department of the Taoiseach. It assists communities to participate fully in local development and in targeting services and resources to those in most need (Area Development Management Ltd, 1995).

The stepwise process described above represents a general model that must be modified to meet local conditions and needs. The objectives of promoting community participation will vary according to the perceptions, expectations and resources of the participants and should be set out unambiguously at the start to avoid unrealistic expectations. It is also essential for subsequent evaluation that the objectives and procedures established for the participation process itself be sufficiently explicit that progress towards their achievement can be accurately measured. It must also be borne in mind that community involvement raises expectations for change and that these will have to be met within the limits of available resources. It is, for example, valuable for a general practice to have a clearer idea of the demographic, epidemiological and sociological characteristics of its population and also to know more of the health perceptions and priorities held by the community. However, the process of obtaining this information constitutes a commitment to respond, and this may not always be in ways that are advantageous to the provider.

To date, three development projects have been implemented in Ireland with community participation in healthcare as a specific objective: a rural poverty programme in North-West Connemara involving a district electoral division of about 800 households, a travellers' health project in West Dublin covering four sites and 180 households, and a community development project in a peri-urban community of Dublin with a population of more than 80,000. In all three projects, a health group was organised within the community, the area health authority agreed to provide administrative support and independent providers co-operated to varying degrees. A university department provided technical support, in the form of expertise and skills training, which was financed from its own budget. These projects are described in published articles and formal reports (Quirke *et al.*, 1994; Eastern Health Board, 1996; Trinity College, 1996). In each case, an information base was established and a needs self-assessment carried out by household survey. The needs assessment results were subject to community prioritisation, and local resources were identified to assist implementation of change. The degree to which they have achieved their stated objectives is to be reviewed in the near future.

By its nature, community participation in healthcare is a difficult process to quantify and evaluate in conventional terms. In the first place, it produces valuable social and economic effects in the community beyond specific improvements in service delivery and health status. These broader effects are equally valid, if more general, outcomes of the development process and should therefore be included in any cost–benefit analysis. Secondly, change achieved by active participation is unique to any given community, so that conventional models for health service research are of limited use in evaluating effectiveness. Research concepts and methods from the domain of sociology and anthropology need to be adapted to measure community gain, in addition to evaluating the more direct benefits to users and providers.

The emerging interest in community participation for healthcare planning in Ireland is driven as much by social and political considerations as by the promise of technical and financial advantage to programme managers. In particular, policies and strategies committed to returning primary healthcare to the community will require active participation by people and power-sharing by statutory agencies if we are to convert rhetoric into reality.

CHAPTER 17

Promoting Health: Thinking through Context

MALCOLM MACLACHLAN

Introduction

This chapter does not attempt a review of health promotion in Ireland. Instead it seeks to highlight some issues which should be of particular concern to those engaged in promoting the health of Irish people. Beginning with a brief historical overview of health promotion, I outline two important challenges to the ways in which we promote health: the well-being of travelling people and how inner city communities have responded to the problem of drug misuse. Focusing on the importance of community involvement, I also review the recent large-scale health promotion project in Kilkenny. The components of the varied contexts in which effective health promotion must take root are also considered, paying particular attention to the influence of poverty, urban–rural differences and how distinctive characteristics of Irish culture should be taken into account. It is argued that while targeted intervention studies are absolutely necessary, the diversity of social and cultural contexts within our society must also be addressed at a broader level, in order to maximise the potential benefits of a health-promoting perspective.

Historical overview

The World Health Organisation (WHO) has powerfully influenced current thinking on health and health promotion. In 1948 WHO defined health as '…a complete state of physical, mental and social well-being and not merely the absence of disease or infirmity'. This definition of health reached beyond the previous simplistic idea that health was the absence of illness – it recognised that health is multidimensional, incorporating physical, mental and social aspects.

However, its emphasis on a state of 'complete' well-being is now also outdated. Increasingly we are acknowledging that health is a relative term. We are all healthy in some respects and unhealthy in other respects. For instance, physically handicapped people can lead active and healthy lives, making valued contributions to society (as long as society provides an environment which does not disable them). At the same time, the very paragons of athletic vitality may be crippled by psychological distress or social pressures.

In 1986 WHO produced a *Charter for Health Promotion* (The Ottawa Charter) which described five key elements:

1. building healthy public policy
2. creating supportive environments
3. strengthening community action
4. developing personal skills
5. reorienting health services.

At the same time as WHO produced this Charter, the Irish Government published *Health – the Wider Dimensions* and *Promoting Health through Public Policy*. Both of these documents recognised the need for resources to be invested in the promotion of health and the prevention of illness, rather than simply responding to the immediate demands of treating illnesses as they arose. The Health Strategy document, *Shaping A Healthier Future* (1994) further highlighted the value of promoting health, and the Department of Health's *A Health Promotion Strategy* (1995) is the most recent and comprehensive articulation of the Irish Government's health-promoting philosophy.

Institutional structures to implement the health promotion philosophy have also evolved over recent years. The Health Promotion Bureau, established in 1975, was replaced by the Health Promotion Unit in 1992. There now also exists an inter-sectoral National Advisory Council on Health Promotion and a Cabinet sub-committee chaired by the Minister of Health and composed of ministers from relevant government departments. The Health Promotion Unit led various institutional developments, one of the most influential being the creation of a Centre for Health Promotion at University College Galway (see Kelleher, 1992). While this centre is a focus for research and training, many other Irish universities, institutions and agencies are also active in health promotion. Some of these activities have been generated through links with Health Boards, all of which now either have or aspire to having health promotion officers.

A Health Promotion Strategy is subtitled *making the healthier choice the easier choice.* In many Irish contexts the healthier choice is far from an easy choice. Nowhere is this more apparent than among Ireland's travelling people. Attempts to assimilate travellers into existing health services have, at times, been culturally insensitive. The health status indicators for travellers continue to be far worse than the population average.

Promoting travellers' health

The Travellers' Health Status Study (Health Research Board, 1987) reported that travellers have more than double the national rate of stillbirths, and infant mortality rates are three times the national average. While having higher death rates than the settled community across the board, travellers have particularly high mortality from metabolic disorders (up to the age of 14), respiratory ailments, congenital problems and accidents. Traveller men live on average 10 years less than settled men, while traveller women live on average 12 years less than settled women. In fact, travellers are only now reaching the life expectancy that settled Irish people reached in the 1940s. *Shaping a Healthier Future* emphasises the principle of equity, explicitly acknowledging that this principle 'imposes a particular obligation upon the health services to pay special attention to geographic areas or population groups (*such as travellers*) where the indicators of health status are below average' (p. 23) (emphasis added). The current Four Year Action Plan (of the Department of Health) has identified traveller health as a priority area, targeting the development of models of traveller participation in health promotion and prevention, the development of health education programmes aimed specifically at travellers, ensuring Health Boards make special arrangements to improve access for travellers to services, creating continuity of care across Health Board areas, and ensuring close liaison with other statutory and voluntary agencies to enable better targeting of services.

Despite these worthy recommendations, relatively little has happened. For many travellers the healthier choice is not only a more difficult choice, but often also one of which they are unaware. In a recent study of travellers' views on family planning services conducted in the Midland Health Board area, only 18% of traveller women had any premarital sex education and only 10% knew at what part of their monthly cycle they were most likely to conceive. However, the danger with such statistics is that they are interpreted by some people as supporting a 'deficit model' of traveller health, i.e. travellers are described by what they lack knowledge of relative to the settled population. Travellers are disparaged as ignorant and at times obstinate. A more promising perspective is one which recognises real differences in the lifestyles and life meanings of members of the settled and travelling communities. These differences have been rightly acknowledged to be *cultural differences* by many commentators (e.g. McCann *et al.*, 1994; MacLaughlin, 1995; MacLachlan, 1996).

The Task Force on the Travelling Community (1995) asserts that travellers are indeed a distinctive cultural group with associated needs and particular health service requirements. The report recommends the development of traveller-specific health services, and argues for the participation of travellers in this venture. In one of the few projects to enact these recommendations, the Eastern Health Board has been collaborating with Pavee Point in order to 'assist in reshaping our health services for the special and unique needs of travellers' (Hickey, 1996). The project was concerned with primary health care for travellers, but it is the use of travellers themselves as the healthcare workers that marks it out as a particularly important and imaginative venture.

The project aimed

1. to establish a model of traveller participation in the promotion of health
2. to develop the skills of traveller women in providing community-based health services
3. to liaise and assist in developing dialogue between travellers and health service providers
4. to highlight gaps in health service delivery to travellers, working towards reducing inequalities that exist in established services (Primary Health Care for Travellers Project, Pavee Point & Eastern Health Board, 1996).

The baseline survey component of the project investigated health-service use, help-seeking behaviour, attitudes to traveller illness and breastfeeding, and suggestions for changing existing health services. Once again a distinctive profile of traveller health arose and was targeted by the training of travellers to become Community Health Workers.

For instance, the Primary Health Care for Travellers Project (1996) reported that over 80% of travellers seek cures from ('non-health professional') healers. The two most common complaints for which healers were consulted were thrush and infectious diseases. However, they were also consulted regarding cases of eczema, arthritis, aches and pains, burns, asthma, depression and other problems. Over 70% of travellers felt that their higher rates of illness were attributable to poor living conditions, and over 50% suggested that health services would be improved by the provision of more appropriate information (i.e. more appropriate to the needs of travellers). Thus, any attempts at promoting the health of travellers through targeting infectious diseases that do not take account of the influence of alternative sources of health information (healers), living conditions or the way in which health information is provided should not be expected to impact on the lives of travelling people.

These first steps towards culturally sensitive health promotion must be followed through and similar projects, taking local circumstances into account, developed as joint ventures between travelling people and health-service providers. Cultural differences profoundly affect health (MacLachlan, 1997), and if we are to provide health choices which are easy choices then we must present those choices in culturally sensitive ways.

Drug misuse and community empowerment

While the health of travellers presents one type of challenge to Irish health promotion, the alarming rise in inner-city drug misuse presents a different type of challenge. Again, it also presents opportunities for new ways of promoting health. The problem of illicit drug use has been increasing, especially in Dublin, since the early 1980s. O'Higgins (1996) reported that 75% of those attending for drug treatment cite heroin as their drug of primary use, and that the majority of these drug misusers are from socially disadvantaged areas. Of particular concern is the proportion of those in treatment drawn from the 15–19-year-old age group, this proportion having doubled from 14.4% to 28% between 1991 and 1994. Comiskey *et al.* (1992) reported that the age at which intravenous drug use began ranged from 11 to 28 years for males and 10 to 30 years for females.

Local authority housing estates in the inner-city and suburban communities are areas in which drug problems are most profound. The Combat Poverty Agency has been active in attempting to highlight how the deprived social context in which people live often primes the conditions for high rates of drug misuse (Frazer, 1996). The government, recognising that the 'drug problem' is increasingly becoming a 'youth problem', and that this is linked to social deprivation, has recommended the targeting of ten areas in Dublin through locally based Partnership Companies (Rabbitte, 1996). Such initiatives are very necessary and very welcome. This is especially so when they incorporate the need for fundamental changes, as is the case with the recent government announcement that the Ballymun area of North Dublin is to be pulled down and rebuilt. However, in rebuilding, either literally or metaphorically, it is important to recognise existing strengths.

The 'drugs siege' mentality which has gripped many housing estates, in conjunction with parents' concern to prevent the (drug) abuse of their children, has spawned a community-based response which has been, at times, quite remarkable. While the problem of drug misuse is clearly a threat to health and welfare, communities' responses to this threat should, in themselves, be recognised for their health-promoting (and not just ill-health-preventing) potential. Over the past few years the Irish press has avidly reported on how these communities have responded to their drug threat.

A newspaper article by Maher written in December 1996 suggested that 'When it came to combating the illicit drug trade, 1996 was a year when the people led and the authorities followed'. The first signs of this were seen during March when residents of Tallaght, angry at the openness and intrusiveness of drug trading and the effects it was having on their youth, started mounting patrols and building huts (from wooden pallets and sheets of plastic) around the housing estates. This allowed residents to keep a 24-hour watch on the activity of drug dealers and to report suspicious car registrations to the Garda, whom they considered only occasional visitors to their estates. The idea of this sort of community response spread across other areas of the inner city and West Dublin. By mid-1996 Dublin was witnessing regular marches protesting against drugs and often culminating in protests outside the homes of those suspected of drug dealing. It seems that the majority of the participants in these marches and protests were ordinary citizens fired by fears for their children's futures. Apart from a couple of TDs and local councillors, constitutional politicians have tended to keep a distance from the anti-drug movement.

Community networks – Coalition of Communities Against Drugs (COCAD) and Inner Cities Organisations Network (ICON) – facilitated communities' responses. Residents' groups set up local treatment centres and then sought funding, contrasting with the sometimes poorly received Health Board initiatives. Popular anti-drugs movements were, at least in part, the impetus behind several important subsequent developments regarding illicit drug use, such as increased policing, increased investment by Eastern Health Board in developing treatment services, and increased research funding through Forbairt's Science and Technology Against Drugs grants.

I have suggested that community reactions to problems of illicit drug use should be seen not simply as a preventive or curative response, but also as a response which has the potential to be actively health-promoting. Antonovsky (1996) has described the concept of a Sense of Coherence (SOC) as being a central mechanism for promoting health. Establishing an SOC requires that people find stressful situations

1. meaningful (in the sense that they are motivated to cope with them)
2. comprehensible (believing that the challenge is understood)
3. manageable (believing that the resources to cope are available to them).

These attributes should not relate to only one source of stress: instead, to be truly health-promoting, they should characterise a particular orientation towards the world, so that a wide variety of life problems are reacted to as meaningful, comprehensive and manageable. Of course, many people live in environments which are demotivating, which do not offer opportunities for fully comprehending the nature of many social problems and which are stripped of the necessary resources to manage life's problems. Indeed, this is the case in many deprived inner-city areas (as well as rural areas).

It is in this impoverished environment that community reactions to problems can provide a vehicle for a sense of coherence. Responding to the threat of drugs in a manner which reflects a social meaning (a threat to youth), a sense of comprehension (seeing that the source of the problem lies with, for example, social deprivation, inadequate policing, sparse treatment facilities and insufficient investment in drug-incompatible pro-social activities), and the belief that the problem can be managed (through the empowerment which individuals experience as part of an active community force) is a community strength which should be recognised and built on when we are thinking of 'rebuilding' our inner cities. The SOC experienced in these community responses has the potential to spread beyond drug problems and be harnessed to confront other serious threats to well-being and to be, in itself, health-promoting.

There is, however, a danger of being over-idealistic about the process by which deprived communities, becoming empowered, can be a vehicle to health promotion. A vehicle can be hijacked, and indeed there are numerous reports of subversive elements infiltrating and in some cases dominating community movements, in order to fulfil their own political or criminal agenda. It would be naïve not to acknowledge this, or to highlight the violence perpetrated in the name of some community groups. This is clearly abhorrent, and ultimately can only undermine a process of *promoting health through social empowerment.*

The vehicle of SOC should not be discarded: the hijacking should be prevented. The best way to prevent the hijacking of community groups by subversive and criminal elements (who take the law into their own hands) is through legitimate government bodies being seen to be effective in enforcing the law, and in facilitating local communities to achieve their aspirations. Community movements should be a vehicle for government to achieve good. This requires a more bottom-up approach than we have at present. It may at times mean inconsistencies across communities, because settings and conditions vary across communities. A stronger community-based approach to creating a SOC out of social adversity could be one of the most promising, exciting and authentic forms of health promotion. This potential can only be realised if government is willing to truly *invest in the people.* Until recently, with few exceptions, this has not been the case.

Investing in community health

Identifying the most effective ways of 'investing in the people' is another challenge for health promotion in Ireland. The Kilkenny

Project is an example of a community health-promotion project that set out to invest in the people. Community-based health promotion projects have, however, generally been top-down: knowledgeable and institutionally empowered professionals have told people what they ought to do to gain better health. Without doubt, some of these projects have been successes. The Karelia project in North Finland during the early 1970s showed significant reduction in deaths from cardiovascular disease, and the subsequent Stanford Three Communities Project in the USA demonstrated that the use of health-promoting media alone could also produce positive changes in people's lifestyles and associated reductions in mortality. More recently, the success of comprehensive health-promotion efforts in Wales has demonstrated what can be achieved through well-resourced projects. However, the ability of health-promotion efforts to induce voluntary behaviour changes has been questioned on empirical and theoretical grounds (e.g. McCormick and Skrabanek, 1988; McKinlay, 1993). In the late 1980s Ireland had its own large-scale community health-promotion project: the Kilkenny Health Project (Shelley, 1992).

In March 1985 a community-based programme for the prevention of coronary heart disease was launched in County Kilkenny (Offaly being a control non-intervention county to be used for comparison). Over £1.8 million pounds was provided by a variety of funding organisations, the major ones including the Department of Health's Health Promotion Unit, the Irish Heart Foundation, the National Lottery, the South Eastern Health Board and the Voluntary Health Insurance Board. The project incorporated the scientific, educational and community expertise of a broad range of people both within County Kilkenny and nationally. The health promotion component of the intervention included an awareness programme (incorporating car stickers, handbills and posters), weekly articles (and competitions) in the *Kilkenny People* newspaper, a weekly slot on Radio Kilkenny, a project newsletter called CATCH (*Community Action Towards Community Health*), videos concerned with healthy eating and the production of project cookery books. There were also group meetings and evening classes to promote the aims of the project. A working party was established promoting health education programmes in post-primary schools, and training was provided to teachers in primary schools. A range of other events concerned with nutrition, oral health and personal development took place. In many ways the Kilkenny Health Project was exemplary in the breadth of its interventions.

It was therefore surprising that when the health of Kilkenny and Offaly residents was compared, there were relatively few important differences between them. For example, although there was a significant reduction in the risk of coronary heart disease, this reduction occurred in both counties and there was no significant difference between them. The possible reasons for the failure of the Kilkenny Health Project to have a greater effect have been discussed elsewhere (e.g. Shelley *et al.*, 1995). These researchers have noted that there were important attitudinal barriers to pro-health behaviour change in Kilkenny. In essence, people had reasons to resist changing their behaviour. Sometimes these reasons may include the failure of health-promotion efforts to 'speak to' the health beliefs of ordinary people. Social constructions of health and illness are increasingly recognised as an important area, for they are the conduits of health practices (Milburn, 1996; Petrie & Weinman, 1997).

It is important not to dismiss the results of the Kilkenny Health Project simply because it did not produce the dramatic results we might have liked. Instead we should consider what other factors might have made a difference. I would suggest that a more 'bottom-up' approach, driven by the social constructions of health and illness extant within the community, may have led to a more meaningful and effective intervention. However, for such an approach to be effective we 'professionals' must be willing to learn from the communities we seek to serve, and in doing so possibly to disempower ourselves. Another aspect of this 'disempowerment' may be the need to recognise that health-promotion initiatives should reach beyond the target of influencing individuals to change their lifestyles and, in addition, address the social settings in which individuals must lead their lives. This means broadening the health dimension to include non-health professionals whose work concerns factors, such as poverty, which constitute the contexts in which people live (Marks, 1996).

The context of health promotion

The 'risk factors and lifestyles' approach to health promotion is perhaps the dominant ethos within Ireland. The Department of Health's *A Health Promotion Strategy* states that 'Much of the current toll of disease and illness of the Irish population is strongly associated with environmental determinants and lifestyles' (p. 22). This document correctly highlights the dangers of alcohol and substance misuse, the importance of healthy nutrition, the value of breastfeeding and the benefits of exercise. It also targets reduction in serum cholesterol and blood pressure, increasing awareness of the proper management of diabetes mellitus, reducing high-risk HIV behaviour, improving the level of oral health, reducing mortality due to accidents and promoting mental health. One could hardly argue with the desirability of these aims, although we may question how the aims are to be achieved. Many initiatives seem to emphasise personal responsibility, i.e. that individuals should become aware of and motivated to engage in healthy behaviours (exercise, nutritional eating, breastfeeding, etc.) and avoid unhealthy behaviours (excessive drinking, smoking, high-risk sexual behaviour, etc.). While it is difficult to imagine effective health promotion without the instilling of some degree of personal responsibility, there is also a danger that we ignore the situational factors which have promoted unhealthy behaviours in the first place.

The traditional biomedical model accords with the idea of identifying 'at risk' individuals and targeting intervention at them. The problem, according to this analysis, lies within the person rather than within the person's environment. Not only does the 'risk factors and lifestyles' approach 'decontextualise' the problem, but it may also lead to a tendency to 'blame the victim' (as has been suggested in the case of travellers). If somebody has AIDS, gets a heart attack or is not breastfeeding, then they are performing the 'wrong' behaviours, they have a 'bad' lifestyle and we may be forgiven for lacking sympathy. The blamed victim may in turn denigrate himself or herself, thus making it difficult to maintain the degree of motivation which is often required to overcome unhealthy behaviours (e.g. smoking). Risk factors also often include non-modifiable influences. For instance, gender, age, genetic inheritance and family background – all of which are 'risk factors' for various disorders – are beyond our control. We should discourage this notion of 'fated victims' by placing more emphasis on behavioural and environmental factors which can be modified.

These shortcomings should not lead us to abandon our attempts to promote healthier lifestyles and reduce risk factors. What they do demand, however, is that this endeavour should not be individuated.

Instead there must be a stronger emphasis on intervention at a broader level. McKinlay (1993) has argued that health promotion is most effective through planned sociopolitical change. For instance, he contrasts the effectiveness of adding 8 cents to US cigarette taxes (with a corresponding decrease of 2 million smokers) with the relative ineffectiveness of campaigns targeting more voluntary methods of cessation. It has been estimated that adding a further 20 cents to cigarette taxes would prevent more than half a million premature deaths in the USA. Doorley (this volume, Chapter 2) notes that in Ireland the taxation of cigarettes has not, however, resulted in significant health gains. Once again this demonstrates the importance of taking the context of intervention into account: the elasticity of demand for health-damaging products, such as cigarettes, alcohol or illegal drugs, is likely to vary not only between different cultures but between different groups within the same culture.

A similar argument can be made regarding the reduction in road fatalities and serious injuries, following the introduction of the mandatory wearing of seat belts, which was observed in the UK but to a much lesser extent in Ireland (European Transport Safety Council, 1996). The key to this difference may be the much lower rate of enforcement and penalising associated with this law in Ireland in comparison to the UK (Fuller, 1997). The analogy of a river is often used to make the argument for contextualising health promotion: people fall into a river and are swept downstream. Our health (illness) services intervene to rescue the drowning victim. Health promotion, which is often practised as disease prevention, aims to make better swimmers of them. However, what we should ask is 'Why are people falling into the river in the first place?'. Health promotion needs to move upstream. Moving upstream means taking account of the broader social and economic factors which influence health. Three such factors relevant to contextualising health promotion in Ireland are poverty, geographic location and cultural experience. These are now briefly considered.

Poverty

Reviewing the literature on the relationship between poverty and health, Najman (1993) states that 'those in the lowest socioeconomic group have mortality rates approximately $1^1/2$ to $2^1/2$ times those experienced by people in the highest socioeconomic group' (p. 158).

Najman talks of an 'inverse socioeconomic status (SES)–mortality gradient' for most causes of death, noting that the strongest effects are found for deaths by accidents, poisoning, violence and diseases of the respiratory system. In the case of children (aged 1–15), those in the lowest social class have five times the death rate of those in the highest social class, and for instances of death from fire, drowning and falls, there is a ten times difference (Blaxter, 1983). While these figures clearly implicate poverty in poor health, the ambiguity of the very term 'poverty' may make it difficult to deal with.

Amid a plethora of income- and class-related definitions of poverty, Najman identifies five categories of person in which a disproportionate number fall below the poverty line. These categories are single parents, the unemployed, the aged, the disabled and racial and ethnic minorities. It is salutary to note that the percentage of Irish people falling into one of these groups – particularly single parents, the disabled and the aged – is likely to increase. This is a useful segmentation of poverty as long as we recognise that member-ship of these segments is more than a 'risk factor': it is a social condition, and it is likely to be disadvantageous because of the way in which social institutions and majority society respond to the needs of people in these segments. In essence, it is society's response to such individuals that is impoverished, not the individuals themselves.

Urban–rural deprivation?

Verheij (1996) has reviewed research on urban–rural variations in health, showing that the assumption of urban living being associated with higher rates of disorder is simplistic. What appears to be crucial is the interaction of urban v. rural location with a number of social and personal factors: '...there seems to be a tendency towards better perceived health in rural areas, but this tendency disappears in many studies when controlling for demographic variables such as gender and age and enabling variables like socioeconomic status' (p. 929). Simple urban–rural distinctions are meaningless unless we examine the ways in which such differences are experienced through other important variables. Certainly in my own clinical experience, while stressors and reactions to them may differ in type, they are not so different in process. After qualifying as a clinical psychologist and moving from an urban to a rural location, I swapped financial brokers' worries about the FTSE and their associated 'tube phobias' for farmers' worries about the lambing and their associated 'mart phobias'. The process and functions of the disorders were similar – only the content was different.

In Ireland we are now facing the prospect of legislation and bureaucracy actually creating disordered rural communities. It is important to emphasise here that it is the communities as entities in their own right that are becoming disordered, and so we should not be surprised to find increased rates of disorder among the inhabitants of these communities. The high rate of suicide in rural as opposed to urban areas is now well documented, as is the increased rate of suicide among young farmers. Rural communities are becoming denuded of their life sources: schools, post offices, Garda stations, public houses and churches are being forced to close in some areas, thus reducing the sense of community and social support which may act as crucial buffers to life's stresses. Recent EU agricultural policies, it has been suggested, will require increased farm sizes and a scale of operation where most of Ireland's small farmers will find their activities unprofitable and unsustainable. There are, of course, many arguments for and against such changes, but leaving these aside for the moment, the implication of such changes for health should also be considered. More than this, we must be proactive in ensuring that structures for promoting health are maintained in such communities. Once again, the importance of health promotion in Ireland being achieved through structural interventions is clear.

Irish culture

Murphy (1996) has argued that 'Forces such as late industrialisation and modernisation, globalisation and individualisation as well as the effects of feminism, are all changing significantly the life contexts of adults and children in Ireland' (p. 74). These 'forces' are undeniable, although the relative strength of them is clearly debatable. It would, however, be a mistake to think that Ireland and Irish cultures are hurtling towards a state of universal sameness. This is an important point, because if it is tacitly assumed that such a trend exists, then it may also be assumed that beliefs, attitudes, practices, etc. in Ireland are the same as elsewhere, and that methods which work elsewhere will necessarily also work here. There are, in fact, many aspects of our experience which have produced a distinctive Irish psyche (Halliday & Coyle, 1994).

Not least among these are factual experiences of colonialism, civil war and terrorism, the influence of the Catholic Church, and Ireland being a small island on the fringes of Europe, yet achieving great literary and artistic fame. On less factual accounts, the Irish have been stereotyped as heavy drinkers, lawless, violent and sexually repressed. In myth and reality, and where the two knit together in everyday experience, being Irish is not *like being* anything else! Health promotion in Ireland, like any other meaningful social intervention, must therefore take account of the particular characteristics, social constructions and institutional exigencies which shape our obvious need for better health.

It is frequently argued (see e.g. Kelleher, 1996) that health promotion should be distinguished by its positive and holistic (as opposed to reductionist) approach and its concern with the social context in which people make health choices. However, for these aspirations to be realised health promoters need to embrace the potential value of communities and cultures (and subcultures) as conduits of health (MacLachlan, 1997). This is being increasingly recognised in mainstream health promotion. Milburn (1996, p. 42) argues that 'there is a need for a more flexible approach to theory building in health promotion. Principally, the need to bring back culture and the failure of existing theory to tap into the richness, complexity and diversity of human experience, argue for a theorising which will reveal those lay structures of thought and behaviour which are integral parts of everyday health-related behaviour.' The need for such theory, and theoretically driven practice, is as strong in Ireland as anywhere else. In aiming to achieve international standards of excellence we must also take account of our own particular problems, opportunities and strengths and how these are woven into the fabric of Irish life. Table 17.1 summarises some of the issues raised in this chapter by casting them as a series of questions, which may help health promoters to *think through* the contexts in which health choices must be made.

Conclusion

This chapter has attempted to highlight critically 'pressure points' for health promotion in Ireland. There are, in fact, many such pressure points, but the two that have been highlighted here – the health of travellers, and inner-city community reactions to drug misuse – suggest

Table 17.1. Questions for contextualising health promotion

---

1. What are the characteristics of the target group?
2. What is the context in which they live?
3. What role might poverty, geographic location, cultural (or subcultural) identity, or other factors, play in influencing health choices?
4. What lifestyle choices are there, and how are these constrained or facilitated by contextual factors?
5. What is the language of health discourse – what are the health beliefs of target group members?
6. How should members of the target group be included in health planning, implementation and evaluation?
7. Which aspects of the target group's cultural or community identity could act as a vehicle for promoting health?
8. What are the structural barriers to group or community empowerment, and what structural changes may facilitate healthier choices?

---

that the social context of health problems must be given much greater attention than has been the case. 'Problem groups' may also have the potential to develop their own solutions. For instance, travellers have trained as healthcare workers and inner-city communities have found (usually positive) ways of empowering their own residents. However, because it is often the context in which people live that is threatening to their health (poverty or rural depopulation, for example), community initiatives alone are insufficient. They must be supported by policies and structures which address the context of people's lives.

In terms of the Ottawa Charter for health promotion, some progress has been made regarding the development of personal skills and reorienting health services. The remaining three components of the Charter have not received sufficient attention: building healthy public policy, creating supportive environments, and strengthening community action. Efforts to encourage individuals to adopt healthy lifestyles must continue and, indeed, increase. In order to make the healthier choice truly the easier choice in Ireland today, health-promotion efforts must incorporate the cultural, community and contextual resources that are available to us.

CHAPTER 18

Towards Patient-Centred Care: Consumer Involvement in Healthcare

Eilish Mc Auliffe

Introduction

> I received an ante-natal appointment for 1.30 p.m. I arrived at the
> outpatient clinic at 1.25 p.m. (by this time all the seats were occupied, as
> heavily pregnant women lined up to be weighed in turn), and queued for
> 10 minutes to be weighed and have a urine sample checked. I then took a
> seat and waited until 1.50 p.m., when I was called into the consultation
> cubicle and told to take my shoes off and sit on the bed. At 2 p.m. I
> overheard a nurse in the corridor say that the consultant would be arriving
> in 10 minutes. At 2.10 p.m. (40 minutes after my scheduled appointment
> time) the consultant entered the consultation cubicle, accompanied by a
> student whom he introduced to me. During the examination the consultant
> asked the student several questions. I was not quite sure whether the
> questions were directed at me or the student. I mentioned to the consultant
> that I was concerned about the possible side-effects of having a fibroid
> removed if it was necessary after the delivery. The consultant asked me
> 'are you a nurse?'. When I replied 'no', the consultant said that the
> procedure was far too complicated to explain it to me, and with this
> comment he left.*

In my opinion, the most concerning issue about this experience is
not that I had been treated badly, but that most people (including
healthcare personnel) would probably feel I had nothing to complain
about. Yet I waited 40 minutes after my scheduled appointment time
(and I was lucky – the block booking system meant that some women

---

* This vignette is derived from personal experience of the public appointment
system at an ante-natal clinic.

arrived at 1.30 p.m. and not were not seen until 3 p.m.), my permission was not sought for the presence of a medical student, and the consultant suggested I did not have the intellect to understand a simple surgical procedure. This is a snapshot of our health service from a patient's perspective. Is this service patient-centred?

This chapter briefly examines the concept of patient-centred care, as well as developments in acknowledging the rights of the consumer in healthcare, particularly in the UK's National Health Service and in the Irish health service. The concept of 'consumers' is explored – who are they, why should we involve them, and how involved do we want them to become? Techniques for involving consumers are discussed and examples provided. The chapter concludes with a brief examination of the pitfalls in undertaking any consumer involvement activity.

Patient-centred care

Patient-centred care has become a very popular concept in recent years, and there is a growing recognition that current health service structures may be hindering the development of a more patient-centred approach to service delivery. The Health Strategy, *Shaping a Healthier Future*, questions both the focus of healthcare

> Many of the services are not sufficiently focused towards specific goals or targets, and it is therefore difficult to assess their effectiveness (p. 10)

and the systems through which healthcare is currently delivered

> to achieve the objective of providing care in an appropriate setting, it is essential that there are effective linkages between the services. Hospitals, general practitioners and other community services should operate as elements of an integrated system within which patients can move freely as their needs dictate. At present, the system is too compartmentalised to permit this flexibility. (p. 26)

The strategy places great importance on the participation of the consumer in healthcare and on improving linkages between services to provide the most appropriate care. Accountability is one of the key principles of the strategy, and emphasis is placed on accountability to the consumers of the service:

> there must also be mechanisms to ensure that those with decision-making powers are adequately accountable to the consumers of the services. (p. 11)

The traditional functional structures, with divisions between medicine, nursing support and administrative activities, with hindsight, seem to have served the needs of the organisation and healthcare staff more adequately than they served the needs of the patient. Although the changes in structures, and particularly hospital structures, vary from country to country, it is commonly recognised that for any new structures to be judged as being effective, the restructuring must result in improvements in patient care. Thus, one of the primary considerations in changing a hospital's structure should be to ensure a more patient-centred approach to service delivery.

The general approach that is emerging is the realignment of services and staff around particular types or groupings of patients or problems. The terminology associated with the restructuring varies from one country to another, with the USA describing the new entities as patient-focused hospitals (Lathrop *et al.*, 1991), Australia organising into direct patient care units or institutes (which are groups of medical specialities) (Braithwaite, 1995) and the UK and Ireland adopting a similar approach to Australia but using the term 'clinical directorates' or, more recently, 'patient care groups' (Eastern Health Board) to describe these direct patient care units. The basic concept is similar in all these systems, and consists simply of establishing mini-hospitals, units or directorates with specific responsibility for managing particular homogeneous groups of patients – all patients with cardiac problems, all oncology patients, etc.

Of course, the real issue is whether such structural changes really do result in a more patient-centred approach. This has proved difficult to measure. Patient-centred care can only be determined a success if patients find it easier to access the services they need. Given that this is the ultimate goal of reorganising the structures of health systems, it would seem logical that patients should at least be consulted, if not involved, in the process. Services can only become truly patient-centred by understanding the perceptions, concerns and expectations of patients/consumers and building the service around this core.

Recognition of the rights of the healthcare consumer

In recent years the public's expectations of healthcare have escalated. The media have played their part in enlightening the public about health services through TV programmes and health columns in national newspapers. Consumers of healthcare are increasingly demanding a higher-quality and more responsive healthcare service. The Department of Health Statement of Strategy (Department of Health, 1997b) identifies one of the principal challenges as 'growing consumer consciousness in healthcare and growing demands and expectations for higher-quality, consumer-oriented services' (p. 10).

Internationally

At the international level, the right of citizens to participate in decisions about healthcare was formally acknowledged in the WHO/ UNICEF Declaration of Alma Ata in 1978. Clause IV sets out the right and duty of people to plan and implement healthcare. Also, one of the underlying principles of WHO's Health for All by the Year 2000 is community participation. The WHO Declaration on the Promotion of Patients' Rights in Europe (WHO, 1994) distinguishes between social rights, e.g. equity of access, and individual rights, e.g. privacy, confidentiality and consent.

In the UK National Health Service

The beginnings of consumerism in the UK National Health Service (NHS) go back to the 1970s. Patient participation groups in general practice have existed in some areas since the early 1970s, and by 1989 there were 306 such groups in England and Wales (Rigge, 1996). In 1974, community health councils were established as public watchdogs of the NHS, with the purpose of representing local communities' interests to the managers of the NHS. The Association of Community Health Councils (CHCs) for England and Wales (ACHCEW) was set up in 1977 to provide research and information to its member CHCs (now a total of 206) and to lobby ministers and the professions on behalf of service users. The College of Health was founded in 1983 in response to the perceived imbalance in power between health professionals and patients. Its role is to provide information to patients to enable them to make 'informed choices' about health services. The Patients' Forum was established in 1988–89 by the National

Consumer Council and the Patients' Association. This consists of a bi-monthly meeting bringing together groups such as Age Concern and the College of Health with the British Medical Association and the Royal College of Nursing.

The NHS produced a national patients' charter, which was followed by a patients' charter for each district. There also exists a patient empowerment group within the NHS Management Executive (NHSME), and a national freephone number for people to ring for information on every aspect of the health service. Consumer organisations, such as the Patients' Association and the College of Health, are invited to the Department of Health to inform ministers of how they perceive changes in terms of the effect on patients.

The Patients' Association was relaunched in 1996 in an attempt to raise its profile and improve its role as the 'organisation which protects patients' rights'. Also in 1996, the NHS Executive launched its Patient Partnership Strategy. Its aim is to work closely with professional training and regulatory bodies to encourage patient partnership in the NHS.

In the Irish Health Service

In Ireland, the report *Health – The Wider Dimensions* (Department of Health, 1986) addressed the importance of mechanisms for 'active consumer feedback and input'. It also recommended that Community Health Committees be established with the objective of providing a formal input for the local community to local decision-making about health matters.

The Hospital Action Plan (Department of Health, 1990b) placed strong emphasis on a consumer orientation in the delivery of health services and called for a hospital code of conduct and a patient feedback mechanism to be introduced in each hospital. The Dublin Hospital Initiative Group (1991) emphasised the importance of consumer satisfaction, and of achieving this through effective quality assurance programmes. Among the recommendations from the Group was that individual appointment times should be given for outpatient clinic appointments.

The *Charter of Rights for Hospital Patients* (Department of Health, 1992b) sets out a number of rights for hospital patients including the right to information, confidentiality, access, redress, courtesy, privacy and individual appointment times. The only right that relates specifically to the principle of choice is the right to refuse to participate in teaching/research.

There has been much scepticism about the Patients' Charter in this country, and angry reactions from some of the health professionals at the fact that no additional resources were allocated to meeting the expectations raised by the charter. A review of the charter, conducted two years after its publication, in the hospitals of one Health Board (Department of Health, 1992b) indicated that only 26% of surveyed hospital patients had heard of the Patients' Charter, while only 10% of those who had heard of it could recall any of the rights mentioned in it. The survey also highlighted the fact that socio-economic status influenced the likelihood of patients being aware of the charter, with non-medical card holders having twice the likelihood of having heard of it. In relation to the recommendations in the charter concerning complaints procedures, the review surveyed six acute hospitals in one Health Board area and found that while four of the hospitals had designated complaints officers, none of them had their complaints procedures displayed for patients to see (O'Donovan & Casey, 1995).

The Ombudsman plays an important role in protecting the rights of the healthcare consumer. Under the 1980 Ombudsman Act, he has statutory jurisdiction over all Health Boards, as well as government departments and local authorities (Wood *et al.*, 1995). The jurisdiction of the Ombudsman, however, does not extend to the exercise of clinical judgement, i.e. the diagnosis, clinical treatment or prognosis of any patient. The Ombudsman acts in response to complaints from members of the public. Such a complaint must fulfil three criteria in order for the Ombudsman to investigate it:

- the action complained of must have been taken in the performance of administrative functions by a body within the jurisdiction of the Ombudsman
- someone must have been adversely affected by the action
- the action must have been contrary to fair or sound administration, i.e. have resulted from maladministration (which could include negligence, carelessness, improper discrimination, undesirable practice or faulty procedures, failure to provide reasonable information or the giving of misleading or inadequate information) (K. Murphy, 1996).

The Irish Patients' Association was established in 1995 as an independent consumer group. Its aim is to 'encourage and assist ongoing developments in quality, safety, availability and cost-effectiveness of all health services to the benefit of all patients' (Irish Patients' Association, 1995).

The Irish Society for Quality in Healthcare was also established in 1995. Its role is to promote quality initiatives in healthcare in Ireland, to generate debate on quality issues and to encourage sharing of experience and expertise in quality management among health agencies.

What is consumerism?

The primary purpose of the recognition of consumers' rights, and of the whole consumerism movement, is to empower consumers by shifting the balance of power from providers to consumers. Consumerism is concerned not just with the recognition but also with the protection of consumers' rights. Epstein (1990) describes the five basic principles of consumerism as:

1. *information* – patients have a right to information about their diagnoses, their prognoses and the treatment options available to them, as well as information on the relative success of the various options and any known side-effects
2. *access* – all citizens should have access to the best available healthcare, regardless of geographical location or socio-economic status
3. *choice* – wherever possible, patients should be involved in the choice of the most appropriate treatment option
4. *redress* – the healthcare system should have in place a procedure which allows patients to complain if they are unhappy with any aspect of their treatment
5. *representation* – patients/consumers should be represented on decision-making and planning bodies.

Berry (1988) identifies three models of consumerism. The first model treats service users as purchasers of services; the second recognises the importance of consultation with users, whose views, according to the model, should be elicited in order to ensure that the service is appropriate to its users. The third model proposes the empowerment of users to facilitate their participation in policy-making.

Who is the healthcare consumer?

Who is the consumer or user in healthcare? A patient is defined as 'a person in receipt of medical care'. However, those who are affected by the healthcare system are not just those people who are in receipt of medical care. Consumers also include the carers or relatives of patients. Indeed, in essence any member of the public – every citizen – is a potential consumer of healthcare. We therefore need to consider the perceptions of the public, if our healthcare system is to be truly responsive to our citizens.

Beresford and Croft (1993) distinguish consumerist and democratic approaches to citizen involvement. Democratic approaches to citizen involvement, they argue, are based on the concept of empowerment and are primarily concerned with finding methods of achieving true participatory democracy, with citizens actively involved in the policy-making process. These democratic approaches aim to empower citizens to critique existing power structures, to raise people's social and political consciousness and incite them to collective action. Consumerist approaches, on the other hand, give priority to the needs of consumers and translate these needs into markets.

If we are to protect the rights of our consumers, it is necessary that we have some mechanism of obtaining feedback from or consulting with those consumers and citizens. There is much debate about whether it is possible to provide equitable health services that adequately meet the needs of the population by consulting only with consumers. One could argue that consumers are the best people to consult with, or involve in planning and delivering health services, since they are the ones with direct experience of the service and may therefore be more able to identify its shortcomings.

However, there is also the problem that, as consumers – particularly if they are regular consumers – they will have a vested interest in the development of services that pertain mainly to their own health problems. This argues for casting the net wider and involving the general public. Of course, every citizen will have their own unique experience of the health services, either directly or indirectly through relatives or friends. None the less, the involvement of citizens rather than just consumers is likely to be more democratic. In some cases, however, the cost of this democratic process may well be prohibitive and the service providers may argue in favour of confining the process to consumers, given that they are a captive audience and there is less expense involved in bringing them together. Perhaps there is no perfect solution and each option has to be evaluated on its merits in terms of the feedback or input required. For example, if a Health Board is attempting to improve communications with cancer patients, it will be more appropriate to involve patients or consumers who are currently receiving treatment. However, if a Health Board is trying to decide where to locate a treatment centre for drugs and alcohol, then obviously the opinion of the wider public will be important.

Why involve the consumer/citizen in healthcare planning and evaluation?

In general, healthcare systems benefit from improved quality of care through the use of consumers' views. A more in-depth understanding of the consumers can lead to a better patient–clinician relationship and indeed increase patient compliance, which in turn leads to a quicker recovery. Consumer participation also creates greater unity among healthcare personnel by keeping personnel more focused on the ultimate goal of caring for the patient or consumer, thus ensuring service delivery is more patient-centred or patient-focused. It helps to improve the public image of the healthcare system, reduces litigation and aids in public accountability. It is also a tool to assist us to monitor progress in the achievement of the outcomes of health and social gain.

A more active level of participation, on the part of the consumer, can benefit the system by enabling consumers to share in the responsibility for priority-setting and decision-making, and this in turn can lead to more efficient resource utilisation. Some healthcare professionals will argue that consumers are not equipped to participate in this manner, because of their lack of knowledge of the technical aspects of healthcare. However, it is not envisaged that consumers alone will set priorities. What is needed is a partnership between healthcare providers (both clinicians and managers) and healthcare consumers, each having an input into the decision-making process. Until this type of dialogue occurs, we cannot expect to succeed in providing patient-centred care.

How do we involve the consumer/citizen?

The methods one chooses to involve the consumer/citizen are to a great extent dependent on the level of involvement desired. At the most basic level, there is the *provision of information* to consumers – information about the services on offer, information about their condition and the treatment they are receiving or are about to receive. To take it a step further, we may wish to enter into *consultation* with our consumers and there are a series of methods and processes to allow us to do this. The choice of method is important if token consultation is to be avoided:

> Handing out tick-in-the-box patient satisfaction questionnaires and then sitting smugly back if the results indicate that most patients are satisfied with the service they have received (as many quantitative methods do) is no substitute for genuine consultation. (Rigge, 1995, p. 12)

Consultation is about seeking the opinions of consumers, and their opinions may be sought on a variety of different aspects of the service. However, consultation does not imply choice for the consumer, and often the problem with consultation is that the feedback received from consumers is not acted on, i.e. is not used to improve the service. To be truly consumer-responsive, a service needs to engage the consumer in *active participation* in the planning and evaluation of health services. In effect, the healthcare planners/providers need to form a *partnership* with the consumer. In order to be effective, this partnership needs to be a long-term partnership with commitment from all parties involved.

The level of involvement which the health service decides to have with its consumers is dependent on a number of factors, including

- the initial impetus for deciding to involve consumers
- the perceived benefits in relation to the amount of effort that needs to be expended
- the level or degree of consensus in relation to the approach or method that is used to involve consumers.

In the NHS, one of the criteria that the purchasing authorities use in deciding on a provider agency to provide services is the level or degree of satisfaction of patients with that particular provider. This puts an onus on the provider to implement a system to measure patient satisfaction in its service. However, what the provider hopes to gain from this exercise is a report stating that there is a high level of satisfaction with the service. For this reason, the provider agency may be tempted to ask questions, or seek opinions of patients, only on aspects of the service which they themselves consider to be of good quality. There is less incentive for the provider to probe into areas of difficulty where the consumer or patient might suggest improvements to the service.

The situation in Ireland is that the Department of Health has recently stipulated that all Health Boards and hospitals should include in their annual report some account of how they are measuring quality assurance in attempting to involve their consumers or patients in the improvement of the service (Department of Health, 1996c). However, the Department did not dictate the level or degree of involvement that the consumer should have in service planning or delivery.

On the other hand, *Shaping a Healthier Future* states clearly that the outcomes of the health system should be health gain and social gain. If health gain and social gain are to be the outcomes by which we measure the performance of our health delivery system, then we cannot ignore the consumer in healthcare. Health gain goes beyond the concept of an improvement in the physical functioning of the patient to include an improvement in the quality of life of the patient, a concept which can only be measured by obtaining the views and opinions of patients themselves. Therefore, a system which measures its performance by the health gain of its patients needs to form a partnership with those patients. The concept of social gain, being much wider than health gain, requires a partnership with the community/catchment population or advocates of this group, who are likely to benefit from health interventions.

Most, if not all, Health Boards consider their mission to be the enhancement of health and social gain for their catchment populations, rather than the narrower goal of health and social gain for the Health Board's patients only. In order to achieve health and social gain for the population, each Health Board will need to make choices about resource utilisation and service prioritisation that are appropriate to its catchment population. Who should make these choices? Should the public have any involvement in such decisions?

In the well-known and controversial experiment conducted in Oregon State in the USA in 1991, public approval was sought for placing limits on some forms of treatment, in order to increase access to healthcare by people previously denied it. This experiment has been the subject of heated international debate. In an evaluation paper, the US Office of Technology Assessment commended the state for its attempts to broaden public input, but criticised the fact that the public meetings held were not representative of the State's population (two-thirds of the participants were healthcare workers) (Congress of the US, 1992).

One of the most common approaches to involving consumers in the UK has been the establishment of community health councils (CHCs) in the mid-1970s. Although the councils vary greatly in their effectiveness and indeed in their remit, recently the appropriateness of the role of the CHCs as public watchdogs has been questioned, and there are some suggestions that they should form closer partnerships with health authorities (Millar, 1996). Among the recommendations made by the recent review of CHC resource allocation and performance management, commissioned by the NHS Executive, is that the CHCs should monitor local health services towards specific projects agreed with their health authority. While the CHCs are keen that their role should be clarified, they maintain that they have to remain independent in order to do their jobs. However, given the variability in the effectiveness of CHCs throughout the UK, it would seem that more stringent performance management may be necessary to improve accountability to the public. It has also been suggested that in some cases it is questionable whether CHC members are true advocates for patients.

In 1991 the Lothian Health Council attempted to overcome some of these problems by establishing a healthcare evaluation team, consisting of council members and independent research professionals (Stevenson & Hegarty, 1994). They then established a joint working group comprising members of this healthcare evaluation team and healthcare professionals who were involved in the service being audited, to oversee the process. This approach proved successful in that it allowed them to ensure that the audit was indeed consumer-led, that an appropriate methodology was chosen for the particular study, that the analysis and recommendations emerging from the study would be policy-relevant and that through the involvement of healthcare staff there would be ongoing involvement in implementing the research and the recommendations.

A similar approach was adopted by the author in a consumer audit of dental services in the Eastern Health Board. A working group consisting of an independent evaluator, healthcare professionals and a consumer representative was established. The role of this working group was to oversee the audit process and to decide on the most appropriate samples and methodologies. A primary aim of this work was to change gradually the composition of the working group, so that eventually it would consist of one representative of the Health Board and seven consumer representatives, who would oversee a continuous service improvement monitoring and feedback loop. Although the originally established working group has fulfilled its function, it is proving difficult to identify consumers (in this case parents of children receiving dental treatment) who are willing to volunteer to work on this committee. None the less, involving the service providers in the planning and detailed design of the study proved invaluable. When health professionals feel some degree of ownership and control of the exercise, the consumer audit process is likely to run much more smoothly and be far more beneficial in terms of preparing the ground for change (Mc Auliffe & MacLachlan, 1992; MacLachlan & Mc Auliffe, 1992).

A novel approach was adopted by Leicester General Hospital in order to obtain patients' views. In 1995 they set out to:

- obtain information from patients similar to that obtained when a friend or relative had experience of the acute care system
- involve managers and other staff who do not normally deal with patients
- capture patients' perceptions in a way which made the findings easy to analyse
- complete the exercise within five months (Thomas, 1996).

They recruited what they call patient 'trackers' through an invitation in the hospital information bulletin. A total of 42 trackers were recruited and these included secretaries, pathology assistants, porters, technicians, human resource advisers and nurses. All the trackers were trained in listening skills and eliciting information. The trackers then approached the patient in the waiting area and introduced themselves to the patient. If the patient agreed to be interviewed, the tracker went ahead and interviewed the patient before they were seen in the clinic. After the patient's appointment with the doctor, the tracker interviewed the patient again and accompanied them to any further tests or X-rays. The observation and discussion were continued in this way. Trackers were also assigned to day-case patients at the beginning of the day, and interviewed them before the procedure and again before discharge. In the case of inpatients, trackers would meet them at least three times during their stay – on admission, soon after treatment and before discharge.

The exercise proved beneficial in several respects. It raised the awareness of the importance of listening to patients. It exposed staff who were not normally involved in patient care to some of the real issues for patients, and very little additional budget was required for the project.

More recently, the citizens' juries approach has been adopted by some health authorities in England and Wales, as a more democratic means of public participation in healthcare decision-making. A citizens' jury brings together a small group of people chosen at random to represent their community. The jurors are provided with relevant information and witnesses whom they may interrogate. Their role is to deliberate among themselves and come to a decision on a matter of healthcare policy. This approach was originally pioneered by the Institute for Public Policy Research (IPPR) in the UK. In 1996 it piloted five juries, all of which addressed health policy questions. The questions considered included, for example, the following.

- Should the public be involved in priority-setting?
- What criteria should be applied to decisions?
- What can be done to improve the quality of life for people with severe and enduring mental illness, carers and their neighbours? (Coote & Lenaghan, 1997)

Early in 1997, the King's Fund sponsored a further three pilot juries in three health authorities (New, 1997). The issues addressed by the juries were: whether the public would accept GP services from nurse practitioners, community pharmacists, or salaried doctors; where to site services for gynaecological cancer; and whether or not to buy chiropractic and osteopathy services for people with back pain. New (1997, p. 3) believes that citizens' juries offer the best of both worlds:

> Power is potentially given to the citizen, but only once proper deliberation has taken place, and after those supporting the various options have been allowed to present their case fully in a carefully managed way. Involving people directly in decision-making may even revitalise interest in community issues and resurrect the notion of the 'active citizen'.

Avoiding the pitfalls

Few of the benefits of partnerships with patients have been realised in Irish Health Boards and hospitals, the primary reason being that consumer involvement activity is mainly focused at the *information/ consultation* phase, and has not as yet moved along the continuum to *active participation* with consumers. Although several consumerism activities are taking place in the Irish healthcare system, they have primarily been focused on hospital patients, with the most popular methodology being the questionnaire survey. These questionnaires tend to focus on issues such as facilities, cleanliness, food and noise level, and rarely ask about relationships with healthcare professionals or, indeed, impressions of clinical care. Some Health Boards have more recently conducted focus groups with particular consumer groups, obtaining more qualitative information on consumers' perceptions on a wide range of issues. Some of these studies have been reported in summary form by the Irish Society for Quality in Healthcare (1997). Another approach which has been adopted to involve consumers is the public meeting. A series of these has been held in different Health Board areas, particularly in relation to issues such as women's health and travellers' health.

   Unfortunately, as experience to date in both the UK and Ireland shows clearly, there is neither a 'one best approach' to involving healthcare consumers nor a foolproof method of ensuring that feedback is acted on. However, even a brief review of the pitfalls warns us that it is worth giving careful consideration to finding the most appropriate approach in any given set of circumstances, and to planning at the outset how the information gained will be used to improve services on an ongoing basis. Therefore, before embarking on a consumer project, managers and other health professionals need to do some careful planning in order to avoid tokenism and ensure that the exercise produces meaningful and worthwhile results. The following are some of the issues that need to be considered.

Why do you want to involve the consumer?

It is important to be clear from the outset as to why you want to involve consumers. In order to achieve this clarity of purpose it may be necessary to interview all the stakeholder groups about their own particular objectives/reasons for requesting or wanting to take part in the exercise. The objectives of different stakeholders may vary from 'wanting to be seen to be taking the views of consumers into account' to 'a genuine desire to form a partnership with consumers and involve them in decision-making'.

Gauging the level of commitment to the exercise is not an easy task, but it is something that needs to be addressed at the outset. For example, if you do not have the support of senior management, i.e. if they are not committed to acting on the views of consumers, you need to be aware of this before you consult your consumers. If this is something you find out after you have engaged the consumers, you may already have raised your consumers' expectations. Failing to deliver on those expectations may damage the relationship between the service providers and their consumers.

Your reasons for involving your consumers will also determine how you involve them. For example, if you simply want cardiac patients to be more informed about what to expect when they are admitted for surgery, you may decide to issue them with an information booklet or video, or invite them to attend an information session. However, if you want to ensure that your facilities for relatives and visitors to the hospital are adequately meeting the needs of these people, you will need to decide on a method of obtaining the views of relatives and visitors on an ongoing basis. This might be done through a comment card, periodic focus group discussions, or an open invitation to submit comments (suggestions and complaints).

Who do you want to involve?

If you are clear about your reasons for wishing to involve consumers, then it will be easier to decide who to involve. Your decision will also be influenced by the resources you have available. Deciding to involve current users, and doing so by issuing a questionnaire to patients in a ward, is a far less expensive option than setting up a citizens' jury or even a series of focus groups. But the less expensive option may not always achieve the desired results. For example, issuing a questionnaire to patients on your maternity ward will not tell you why 40% of expectant women in your catchment area opt to attend the private hospital up the road rather than attending your hospital. Equally, conducting focus group discussions with elderly people who have recently been discharged will not allow you to obtain sufficient information to plan a respite service for the elderly.

When *do you want to involve them?*

The most common approach is to involve consumers when the service provider wants an answer to the question 'How are we doing?', i.e. in the evaluation of the service. If a manager wants the consumers of the service to participate actively as true partners in the planning and delivery of the service, then it is essential to involve the consumers/ citizens in the complete process from the needs assessment to planning the service and setting standards, to monitoring and evaluating.

Another important issue is deciding at what point in the patient/ consumer's path through the service you involve them. If their involvement is sought prior to admission/appointment, it is important to be aware of the 'vulnerability factor', i.e. the possibility that some consumers/patients will be concerned that if they voice negative opinions about the service or the staff, this will impact negatively on their subsequent treatment. In addition to this there is the vulnerability and sometimes anxiety that accompanies illness, both of which make it difficult for the patient/consumer to participate actively. Involvement of consumers immediately after discharge may seem like a better option, but even then there can be interference, particularly in the form of the 'gratitude factor': i.e. the patient/consumer is so delighted to be well again that he/she is very grateful to the service and its providers, and may as a result paint an overly rosy picture of his/her experience in hospital. One might attempt to overcome this factor by delaying the contact until several weeks or months after discharge. By this time the gratitude factor may well have faded, but, most likely, so will the memory of the time in hospital. All these issues need to be carefully considered when one is deciding on the most appropriate time to involve consumers.

Where *will you involve the consumer?*

Context is an important consideration in any interaction with consumers. Again, the vulnerability factor can bias responses if a patient is interviewed in their hospital bed or even in an outpatient clinic while waiting for their appointment. However, the alternative of interviewing patients/consumers in their own homes can be costly and time-consuming. Feedback is less likely to be biased by these factors if the consultation or interaction takes place in a neutral and non-threatening environment. Focus group discussions and public meetings on healthcare issues are often held in community halls or hotel function rooms. Hotels are also a favoured venue for citizens' juries, as the participants may need several days to deliberate before reaching a decision, during which time they need to be sheltered from external influences and possible interference by interested parties.

Another aspect of context, which needs to be carefully considered, is the person or group who will interview, consult with, or involve the consumer. If a nurse/doctor approaches a patient in a hospital bed to seek opinions on his/her perceptions of the staff, it is unlikely that the patient will be completely honest (with the exception of the person who is completely satisfied with his/her treatment and genuinely has no complaint). As a general rule, it is better not to choose staff who are delivering a service to seek opinions on their own service. It may be more appropriate to use staff in other service areas, but they will need training in listening skills, interviewing, facilitating focus group discussions or whatever methodology is to be used. External researchers or management consultants may be more appropriate in large-scale projects or where objectivity or credibility becomes an issue among staff within the service.

How will you involve the consumer?

The range of techniques available for involving consumers is constantly expanding. The important thing is not to insist on using the latest or most popular of these. Instead, one needs to weigh the advantages and disadvantages of each technique in any given situation, and opt for the one (or more) most appropriate to that situation.

Questionnaire surveys are useful if you want to collect quantitative data from a large sample. They also have the advantage of being less costly and time-consuming than interviewing. If a questionnaire is to elicit the issues which are of importance to the consumer, great care must be taken in its design. Unfortunately, this does not always happen, and as a result many questionnaires reflect what is important to the organisation or the researcher rather than to the consumer. Interviews may allow more latitude to the consumer in expressing his/her views, but are costly and time-consuming to administer. Focus group discussions and public meetings are useful for collecting qualitative data, but without rigorous sampling methodology can be very unrepresentative. Another useful technique (which has been around since 1959) for collecting qualitative data is critical incidents

303

technique. Complaints systems are a useful method of obtaining feedback, but because of the negative focus can generate defensiveness, rather than the desire to change or improve, among healthcare professionals. Citizens' juries are perceived to be more democratic than other methods, but are expensive and time-consuming. Other methods such as trackers (described above), mystery clients or comment cards can prove useful in certain situations.

Conclusion

Although much is being done to obtain feedback from healthcare consumers, there are further challenges to be addressed in encouraging the active participation of the Irish public in healthcare. Despite the recommendations in *Shaping a Healthier Future* that we be more accountable to our consumers, we continue to develop health strategies and service plans without any real involvement of the public. To encourage the re-emergence of the 'active citizen', we need to create an environment and a system which enables the public to question continually the adherence of clinicians, policy-makers and managers to 'well-proven' methods of practice. Consumers do not need to understand the complexity of treatment procedures in order to make an informed choice. Instead, healthcare professionals need to be able to explain and predict possible outcomes in layperson's terms. Managers and clinicians need to demonstrate their commitment to the practice of community participation in healthcare.

A national effort to encourage the involvement of citizens in healthcare planning and decision-making is needed. This necessitates a co-ordinated proactive approach. While it is recognised that the Office of the Ombudsman plays an important role in redress for healthcare users, by its nature and remit it can only respond to problems retrospectively and make recommendations for how such problems might be avoided in the future. If our healthcare system is to become more patient-centred, it will require a body or commission that will play an active role in shaping practice towards a more patient-centred approach. What is needed, then, is a type of 'nurturing watchdog'. Although at first glance this may seem like a contradiction in terms, it is possible for one body to perform the two roles, i.e. promoting good practice while also preventing bad practice. In order for this model to work, it would be necessary for such a body to develop close working relationships with the Health Boards and to work with them on a daily basis auditing current practice, drawing comparisons with national practice and piloting models of citizen involvement. It would also play a key role in assisting Health Boards to put into practice the recommendations of the Office of the Ombudsman and to build partnerships with users and citizens. The office would need to have research and project management expertise as well as the expertise required to encourage public involvement and the involvement of health professionals in its activities.

Shaping a Healthier Future addressed the need for a reorientation of the health services, and identified the three dimensions of this reorientation as the *services*, the *framework*, and the *participants*. Progress has been made in focusing the services on health and social gain, particularly since the establishment of the Office for Health Gain. The reorientation of the framework to provide for more decision-making and accountability at regional level has been partly addressed by the recent accountability legislation (the Health (Amendment) Act 1996), by the plans to restructure the new health authorities, and particularly by the Task Force on the Eastern Regional Health Authority (1997). The Department of Health now needs to turn its attention to those participants whose future health will be influenced by these changes. It needs to ensure that Health Boards and hospitals are encouraging citizens to take an active role in shaping a healthier future for the communities they live in.

References and Further Reading

Adirondack, S. (1992) *Just About Managing.* London Voluntary Service Council, London.

Allen, D. (1995) Doctors in management or the revenge of the conquered: the role of management development for doctors. *Journal of Management in Medicine* 9 (4), 44–50.

Antonovsky, A. (1996) The salutogenic model as a theory to guide health promotion. *Health Promotion International* 11 (1), 11–18.

Area Development Management Ltd (1995) *Integrated Local Development Handbook.* Dublin.

Association for Public Health (1997) *Sustaining the Public's Health.* The Manifesto of the Association for Public Health, London.

Audit Commission (1991) *The Virtue of Patients: Making the Best Use of Ward Nursing Resources.* HMSO, London.

Audit Commission (1992) *Making Time for Patients: a Handbook for Ward Sisters and their Managers.* HMSO, London.

Avan, L. (1986) Preface. In A. de la Salle & A. Maurice, *Déracinement et Enracinement des Personnes Handicapées.* CTNERHI, Paris.

Ball, J.A., Hurst, K., Booth, M.R. & Franklin, R. (1989) *Report of the Mersey Region Project on Assessment of Nurse Staffing and Support Worker Requirements for Acute General Hospitals.* Mersey Regional Health Authority and Nuffield Institute of Health Services Studies, Liverpool.

Barnardos (1996) *Disabled People in Britain and Discrimination: a Case for Anti-discrimination Legislation.* Hurst, London.

Barnardos (1997) *If Not Now, When?* Barnardos, Dublin.

Barnes, C. (1992) *Disabled People in Britain and Discrimination: a Case for Anti-discrimination Legislation.* Hurst, London.

Barrington, R. (1987) *Health, Medicine and Politics in Ireland 1900–1970.* Institute of Public Administration, Dublin.

Barton, V. (1993) National casemix project. *Health Services News* 5 (2), May, 16.

Bauer-Scott, G. (1992) *Harvard Business School Review.*

Benner, P. & Wrubel, J. (1993) *The Primacy of Caring: Stress and Coping in Health and Illness.* Addison Wesley, New York.

Beresford, P. & Croft, S. (1993) *Citizen Involvement: a Practical Guide for Change.* Macmillan, London.

Bernard, L.A. & Walsh, M. (1995) *Leadership: the Key to Professionalization of Nursing.* Mosby, London.

Berry, L. (1988) The rhetoric of consumerism and the exclusion of community. *Community Development Journal* 23 (4), 266–272.

Blaxter, M. (1983) Children still suffer from social class. *The Practitioner* 227, 303–305.

An Bord Altranais (1994) *The Future of Nurse Education and Training.* Dublin.

Boufford, J.I. (ed.) (1994) *Doctors as Managers of Clinical Resources.* King's Fund College, London.

Brady, M. (1994) Working paper on management development for doctors in Ireland. In Boufford, J.I. (ed.), *Doctors as Managers of Clinical Resources*, 90–109. King's Fund College, London.

Braithwaite, J. (1995) Organizational change, patient-focused care: an Australian perspective. *Health Services Management Research* 8 (3), Aug., 172–185.

Brechin, A. & Swain, J. (1987) *Changing Relationships: Shared Action Planning with People with a Mental Handicap.* Harper & Row, London.

Brown, S. (1996) Developments in community care for elderly people. *Administration* 44 (3).

Browne, M. (1992) *Co-ordinating Services for the Elderly at Local Level: Swimming Against the Tide.* National Council for the Elderly, Dublin.

Bryson, J. (1988) *Strategic Planning for Public and Non-Profit Organisations. A Guide to Strengthening and Sustaining Organisational Achievement.* Jossey-Bass, San Francisco, CA.

Buchan, J. & Ball, J. (1991) *Caring Costs: Nursing Costs.* Institute of Manpower Studies, Brighton.

Burgoyne, J. & Lorbiecki, A. (1993) Clinicians into management: the experience in context. *Health Services Management Research* 6 (4), 248–259.

Burns, J.M. (1978) *Leadership*. Harper & Row, New York.

Butler, F. (1981) Voluntary inaction. *Community Care*, 19 February.

Caiden, E.G. (1988) The problem of ensuring the public accountability of public officials. *Public Service Accountability: a Comparative Prospective*. Cover, West Hartford, CT.

Canadian Council on Health Services Accreditation (1995) *Standards for Acute Care Organisations*. Ottawa.

Carver, J. (1990) *Boards that Make a Difference*. Jossey-Bass, San Francisco, CA.

Catholic Truth Society (1931) *Quadragesimo Anno*. Encyclical letter of Pope Pius XI. London.

Centenary Health Centre (1992) *By-laws, 1992*. Scarborough, Ontario.

Centers for Disease Control (1997) Editorial note. *MMWR* 46 (24).

Chang, A.M. (1995) Role determination in nursing: implications for service provision. *Journal of Nursing Management* 3, 25–34.

Cole, G.A. (1993) *Management: Theory and Practice*. DP Publications, London.

College of Speech and Language Therapists (1991) *Communicating Quality: Professional Standards for Speech and Language Therapists*. London.

Comiskey, C.M., Ruskin, H.J. & Wood, A.D. (1992) *Mathematical Models for the Transmission Dynamics of HIV in Ireland*. Report for the AIDS Fund, Dublin City University.

Commission on Health Funding (1989) *Report of the Commission on Health Funding*. Stationery Office, Dublin.

Commission on the Status of People with Disabilities (1994) *Family and Personal Support*, working paper. Dublin.

Commission on the Status of People with Disabilities (1995) *Final Report*. Working Group on the Rights of People with Disabilities, Dublin.

Commission on the Status of People with Disabilities (1996a) *The Health Report*, working paper. Dublin.

Commission on the Status of People with Disabilities (1996b) *A Strategy for Equality*. Report of the Commission on the Status of People with Disabilities, Dublin.

Committee on Standards in Public Life (Nolan Committee) (1995) *Standards in Public Life: First Report of the Committee*. HMSO, London.

Congregation for the Doctrine of the Faith (1986) *Instruction on*

Christian Freedom and Liberation. Catholic Truth Society, London.

Congress of the US (1992) *Evaluation of the Oregon Medicaid Proposal: Summary.* Office of Technology Assessment, Washington, DC.

Connell, Archbishop D. (1996) Address at Annual General Meeting of Mater Hospital, 3 September.

Co-ordinating Group of Secretaries (1996) *Delivering Better Government – Second Report to Government of the Co-Ordinating Group of Secretaries. A Programme of Change for the Irish Civil Service.* Stationery Office, Dublin.

Coote, A. & Lenaghan, J. (1997) *Citizens' Juries: Theory into Practice.* Institute for Public Policy Research, London.

Costain, D. (ed.) (1990) *The Future of Acute Services – Doctors as Managers.* King's Fund Centre, London.

Council for Social Welfare (1991) *Submission to the Department of Social Welfare on Proposed Charter for Voluntary Social Services.* Dublin.

Covey, S.R., Merrill, A.R. & Merrill, R.R. (1994) *First Things First.* Simon and Schuster, London.

Cowling, A. & Mailer, C. (eds) (1990) *Managing Human Resources.* Arnold, London.

Cullen, C. (1988) A review of staff training: the emperor's old clothes. *Irish Journal Of Psychology* 9 (2).

Currin, B. (1992) Summing up: civil society organisations in emerging democracies. *Conference of Institute of International Education and Danish Centre for Human Rights on the Role of Voluntary Organisations in Emerging Democracies: Experience and Strategies in Eastern and Central Europe and in South Africa,* Prague. Internet address: http://wn.apc.org/SAIE/civilsoc/

Daft, R.L. (1992) *Organizational Theory and Design,* 4th edn. West Publishing Company, St Paul, MN.

Davidson, A. (1990) General management at district level. In Costain, D. (ed.) *The Future of Acute Services – Doctors as Managers.* King's Fund Centre, London.

Deakin, N. (1996) The devils in the detail: some reflections on contracting for social care by voluntary organisations. *Social Policy and Administration* 30 (1), 20–38.

Deakin, N., Davis, A. & Thomas, N. (1995) *Public Welfare Services and Social Exclusion: the Development of Consumer-oriented initiatives in the European Union.* Office for Official Publications of the European Communities, Luxembourg.

Deal, T. & Kennedy, A.A. (1982). *Corporate Culture.* Addison Wesley, Reading, MA.

Declaration of Alma Ata (1978) *International Conference on Primary Health Care,* USSR, 6–12 September.

Department of the Environment (1987) *Barrington Report.* Stationery Office, Dublin.

Department of Health (1986) *Health – the Wider Dimensions.* Stationery Office, Dublin.

Department of Health (1990a) *The Years Ahead: a Policy For The Elderly.* Stationery Office, Dublin.

Department of Health (1990b) *Hospital Action Plan.* Stationery Office, Dublin.

Department of Health (1991) *The Efficiency Review of Acute Hospitals* (Fox Report). Stationery Office, Dublin.

Department of Health (1992a) *Green Paper on Mental Health.* Stationery Office, Dublin.

Department of Health (1992b) *A Charter of Rights for Hospital Patients.* Stationery Office, Dublin.

Department of Health (1994) *Shaping a Healthier Future – A Strategy for Effective Healthcare in the 1990s.* Stationery Office, Dublin.

Department of Health (1995a) *Developing a Policy for Women's Health.* Stationery Office, Dublin.

Department of Health (1995b) *The Health Promotion Strategy – Making the Healthier Choice the Easier Choice.* Stationery Office, Dublin.

Department of Health (1996a) *National Cancer Strategy.* Stationery Office, Dublin.

Department of Health (1996b) *National Alcohol Policy.* Stationery Office, Dublin.

Department of Health (1996c) *Annual Letter of Allocation to Health Service Agencies.* 23 December, Dublin.

Department of Health (1997a). *Smoking and Drinking among Young People in Ireland.* Stationery Office, Dublin.

Department of Health (1997b) *Statement of Strategy.* Stationery Office, Dublin.

Department of Health (London) (1995) *The Health of the Nation. Variation in Health. What Can the Department of Health and the NHS Do?* A report produced by the Variations Sub-Group of the Chief Medical Officer's Health of the Nation Working Group.

Disken, S., Dixon, M., Halpern, S. & Shocket, G. (1990) *Models of*

Clinical Management. Institute of Health Services Management, London.

Dixon, M. & Baker, A. (1996) *Management Development Strategy in the Health and Personal Social Services in Ireland Report.* Department of Health, Dublin.

Doherty, D. (1996) Child care and protection: protecting the children – supporting their service providers. 'Protecting Irish children; investigation, protection & welfare', special issue, *Administration* 44 (2), summer.

Drucker, F.P. (1973) *Management: Tasks, Responsibilities, Practices.* Heinemann, London.

Drucker, F.P. (1994) Six priorities for change. *The Atlantic Monthly,* November.

Dublin Hospital Initiative Group (1990, 1991) *Reports of the Dublin Hospital Initiative Group* (four reports). Kennedy, D. (Chairman). Department of Health, Dublin.

Duffield, C. (1991) Maintaining competence for first-line nurse managers: an evaluation of the use of the literature. *Journal of Advanced Nursing* 16, 55–62.

Dutt, A.K. & Costa, F.J. (1985) *Public Planning in the Netherlands.* Oxford University Press, Oxford.

Eastern Health Board (1991) *Towards Agreement: a Way Forward for Voluntary Organisations and the Eastern Health Board.* Unpublished report, Dublin.

Eastern Health Board (1996) *Primary Healthcare for Travellers.* Project report, Dublin.

Edwardson, S.R. & Giovannetti, P.B. (1992) Nursing workload measurement systems. In Werley, H. & Fitzpatrick, J. (eds) *Annual Review of Nursing Research.* Springer, New York.

Epstein, J. (1990) *Public Services: Working for the Consumer.* Review for the European Foundation for the Improvement of Living and Working Conditions. Office for Official Publications of the European Communities, Luxembourg.

European Communities (1992) *Treaty on European Union.* Office for Official Publications of the European Communities, Luxembourg.

European Transport Safety Council (1996) *Seat Belts and Child Restraints: Increasing Use and Optimising Performance.* ETSC, Brussels.

Faughnan, P. (1990) Voluntary organisations in the social services field. *Conference on Partners in Progress: the Role of NGOs,* Galway.

Faughnan, P. & Kelleher, P. (1993) *The Voluntary Sector and the State.* Conference of Major Religious Superiors, Dublin.

Fiedler, B. (1988) *Living Options Lottery.* Prince of Wales' Advisory Group on Disability, London.

Fiedler, B. (1993) *Getting Results: Unlocking Community Care in Partnership with Disabled People.* Living Options Partnership, London.

Fiedler, B. & Twitchin, D. (1992) *Achieving User Participation: Planning Services for People with Severe Physical and Sensory Disabilities.* Prince of Wales' Advisory Group on Disability and the King's Fund Centre, London.

Fitzgerald, A. & Lynch, F. (1998) Casemix measurement: assessing the impact in Irish acute hospitals. *Administration* 46 (1), spring, 29–54.

Fitzgerald, L. & Sturt, J. (1996) Clinicians into management: on the change agenda or not? *Health Services Management Research* 5 (2), 137–146.

Fitzpatrick, J., Kerr, M., Saba, V., Hoskins, L., Hurley, M., Mills, N., Rottkamp, B., Warren, J. & Carpenito, L. (1989) Nursing diagnosis: translating nursing diagnosis into ICD codes. *American Journal of Nursing,* April, 493–495.

Fitzpatrick, L. *et al.* (1995) *Alternative Acute Care – a Study in Mental Health Care.* Mid-Western Health Board.

Frazer, H. (1996) *Submission to Government Ministerial Task Force on Measures to Reduce Demand for Drugs.* Combat Poverty Agency, Dublin.

Fuller, F. (1997) Personal communication to M. MacLachlan.

Gagne, R.C. (1996) Accountability & public administration. *Canadian Public Administration* 39 (2).

Gardner, J.W. (1986) *The Nature of Leadership: Introductory Considerations.* Independent Sector, Washington, DC.

Garfink, C.M., Kirby, K.K. & Backman, S.S. (1991). The university hospital nurse extender program. *Journal of Nursing Administration* 21 (4), 26–31.

Gatrell, J. & White, T. (1996) Doctors and management: the development dilemma. *Journal of Management in Medicine* 10 (2), 6–12.

Gilligan, R. (1991) *Irish Child Care Services Policy, Practice and Provision.* Institute of Public Administration, Dublin.

Green, D.G. (1986) *Challenge to the NHS: a Study of Competition in American Health Care and the Lessons for Britain.* Institute of Economic Affairs, London.

Gunnigle, P. & Flood, P. (1990) *Personnel Management in Ireland: Practice, Trends, Developments.* Gill & Macmillan, Dublin.

Halliday, A. & Coyle, K. (eds) (1994) The Irish psyche. Special issue, *Irish Journal of Psychology* 15 (2,3), 243–507.

Ham, C. & Hunter, D.J. (1988) *Managing Clinical Activity in the NHS.* King's Fund Institute, London.

Handy, C. (1988) *Understanding Voluntary Organisations.* Penguin, London.

Hantrais, L. (1995) *Social Policy in the European Union.* Macmillan, London.

Harrison, J. (1993) Medical responsibilities to disabled people. In J. Swain *et al.* (eds), *Disabling Barriers – Enabling Environments.* Sage, London.

Health Promotion Unit (1996) *A National Survey of Involvement in Sport and Physical Activity.* Department of Health. Stationery Office, Dublin.

Health Promotion Unit (1991) *Nutrition Health Promotion – Framework for Action.* Department of Health. Stationery Office, Dublin.

Health Research Board (1987) *Travellers' Health Status Study: Vital Statistics of Travelling People.* HRB, Dublin.

Hederman, M. (1995) *Report of the Expert Group on the Blood Transfusion Service Board* (Department of Health). Stationery Office, Dublin.

Hensey, B. (1988) *The Health Services of Ireland.* Institute of Public Administration, Dublin.

Hensher, M. & Werneke, U. (1995) Restructuring hospitals. *European Health Care Reforms Workshop,* December.

Hickey, K.J. (1996) Foreword. *Primary Health Care for Travellers Project.* Pavee Point & Eastern Health Board, Dublin.

Holland, W.W. (1991, 1993) *European Community Atlas of Avoidable Deaths,* volumes 1 (1991) and 2 (1993). Oxford University Press.

Holloman, C.R. (1985). Headship versus leadership. *Business and Economic Review,* Jan.–Mar., 35–37.

Horsley, S., Roberts, E., Barwick, D., Barrow, S. & Allen, D. (1996) Recent trends, future needs: management training for consultants. *Journal of Management in Medicine* 10 (2), 47–53.

Hospital Commission (1933–1947) *Reports 1–7 of The Hospital Commission*. Department of Health, Dublin.

Hunt, S. (1990) Building alliances. *Health Promotion International* 5 (3), 79–185.

Hurley, J. (1995) S.M.I. in the public sector in Ireland – challenges and imperatives for top managers. *IPA Public Finance Conference*.

Inions, N.J. (1990) *Privilege & Quality Assurance: the Issues for Canadian Hospitals*. Canadian Hospital Association Press, Ottawa.

Institute of Public Administration (1995). *Strategic Management: the Implementation Challenge*. Dublin.

Irish Heart Foundation (1994) *Happy Heart National Survey. A Report on Health Behaviours in Ireland*.

Irish Matrons' Association (1995) *Irish Nurse Management – the Way Forward*. IMA, Dublin.

Irish Patients' Association (1995) *Putting Patients First. Information for Members*. Dublin.

Irish Society for Quality in Healthcare (1997) *Quality Initiatives in Irish Healthcare*. ISQHC, Limerick.

Irish Times (1997) Social disability. Leading article, 7 January.

Jaco, P.R., Price, S.A. & Davidson, A.M. (1994). The nurse executive in the public sector: responsibilities, activities & characteristics. *Journal of Nursing Administration* 24 (3), 55–62.

Jaffro, G. (1996) The changing nature of Irish voluntary social service organisations. *International Journal of Public Sector Management* 9 (7), 55–59.

Jaques, E. (1990) *Requisite Organization: the CEO's Guide to Creative Structure & Leadership*. Cason Hall, Arlington, VA.

Jaques, E. & Clement, S.D. (1991). *Executive Leadership*. Cason Hall, Arlington, VA.

Jarman, B. (1983) Identification of underprivileged areas. *British Medical Journal* 286, 1705–1708.

Johnson, N. (1987) *The Welfare State in Transition: the Theory and Practice of Welfare Pluralism*. Wheatsheaf, Brighton.

Johnson, Z. & Dack, P. (1989) Small area mortality patterns. *Irish Medical Journal* 82 (3), 105–108.

Johnson, Z., Dack, P. & Fogarty, J. (1994) Small area analysis of low birthweight patterns in Dublin. *Irish Medical Journal* 87 (6), 176–177.

Johnson, Z., Jennings, S., Fogarty, J., Johnson, H., Lyons, R., Doorley, P. & Hynes, M. (1991) Behavioural risk factors among young adults in small areas with high mortality versus those in lower mortality areas. *International Journal of Epidemiology* 20 (4), 989–996.

Johnson, Z. & Lyons, R. (1993) Socio-economic factors and mortality in small areas. *Irish Medical Journal* 86 (2), 60–62.

Journal of Health Gain (1997) Issue 1, March. Office for Health Gain.

Joyce, L. & Kenefick, D. (1997) Health Boards as learning organisations: implications for healthcare management development. *Administration* 45 (1), spring.

Kafka, F. (1988) *The Trial.* Schocken Books, New York.

Kelleher, C. (1992) Promoting our health in Ireland. In C. Kelleher (ed.), *The Future for Health Promotion.* Centre for Health Promotion Studies, University College Galway.

Kelleher, C. (1996) Education and training in health promotion: theory and methods. *Health Promotion International* 11 (1), 47–53.

Kernaghan, K. & Langford, J. (1990) *The Responsible Public Servant.* The Institute for Research on Public Policy & The Institute of Public Administration of Canada, Toronto.

Kieran, P. (1988) Community care supports families? In R. McConkey & P. McGinley (eds), *Concepts and Controversies in Services for People with Mental Handicap.* Brothers of Charity Services, Galway; St Michael's House, Dublin.

Kilkenny Health Project (1992) *The Kilkenny Health Project 1985–1992.*

Kramer, M. (1990) The magnet hospitals: excellence revisited. *Journal of Nursing Administration* 20 (9), 35–44.

Lathlean, J. (1988) *Research in Action: Developing the Role of the Ward Sister.* King's Fund, London.

Lathrop, J.P., Seufert, G.E., MacDonald, R.J. & Martin, S.B. (1991) The patient-focused hospital: a patient care concept. *Journal of the Society for Health Systems* 3 (2), 33–50.

Leahy, A., Wiley, M., Sharkey, M. & Bouchier-Hayes, D. (1997) *Implementing Surgical Audit.* RCSI, Dublin.

Leane, M. & Powell, F.W. (1995) *Towards Independence – a Quality of Life Study of Longstay Psychiatric Patients Returned to Community Living in Waterford, Eire.* University College Cork.

Lundborg, L.B. (1982) What is leadership? *Journal of Nursing*

Administration, May, 22–32.

Lundstrom, F. & McKeown, K. (1994) *Home Help Services for Elderly People in Ireland.* National Council for the Elderly, Dublin.

Mc Auliffe, E. & MacLachlan, M. (1992) Clinicians' resistance to consumer satisfaction surveys: what they never tell you. *Journal of Management in Medicine* 6 (3), 47–51.

McCann, M., O Siochain, S. & Ruane, J. (1994) *Irish Travellers: Culture and Ethnicity.* Institute of Irish Studies, Queen's University Press, Belfast.

McCarthy, G. (1993a) The future of Irish nursing, Part 1. *World of Irish Nursing,* Jul./Aug., 10–12.

McCarthy, G. (1993b) The future of Irish nursing, Part 2. *World of Irish Nursing,* Sept./Oct., 13–16.

McCloskey, J. & Molen, M. (1987) Leadership in nursing. *Annual Review of Nursing Research* 5, 177–202.

McConkey, R. (ed.) (1994) *Innovations in Educating Communities about Learning Disabilities.* Lisieux Hall, Chorley.

McCormack, B. (1988) Voluntary fundraising: a disservice to people with mental handicap. In R. McConkey & P. McGinley (eds), *Concepts and Controversies in Services for People with Mental Handicap.* Brothers of Charity Services, Galway; St Michael's House, Dublin.

McCormick, J. & Skrabanek, P. (1988) Coronary heart disease is not preventable by population interventions. *The Lancet,* 839–842.

McDaid, P. (1988) Issues in planning of a mental handicap service. In R. McConkey & P. McGinley (eds), *Concepts and Controversies in Services for People with Mental Handicap.* Brothers of Charity Services, Galway; St Michael's House, Dublin.

McGowan, C. (1996) A long way from home. *Health Services Journal,* April.

MacIntyre, A. (1985) *After Virtue: a Study of Moral Theory.* Duckworths, London.

McKevitt, D. (1990) *Health Care Policy in Ireland.* Hibernian University Press, Cork.

McKevitt, D. (1996) Strategic management in the Irish Civil Service: Prometheus unbound or phoenix redux. *Administration* 43 (4), winter, 34–50.

McKevitt, D. (1998) *Managing Core Public Services.* Basil Blackwell, Oxford.

McKevitt, D. & Lawton, A. (1996) The manager, the citizen, the politician and performance measures, *Public Money and Management* 16 (3), 49–55.

McKinlay, J.B. (1993) The promotion of health through planned sociopolitical change: challenges for research and policy. *Social Science and Medicine* 36 (2), 109–117.

MacLachlan, M. (1996) Culture sensitive health promotion in Ireland. *Annual Conference of the Psychological Society of Ireland,* Waterford, 7–10 November.

MacLachlan, M. & Mc Auliffe, E. (1992) Overcoming clinicians' resistance to consumer satisfaction surveys. *Journal of Management in Medicine* 6 (3), 52–56.

MacLachlan, M. (1997) *Culture and Health.* Wiley, Chichester.

MacLaughlin, J. (1995) *Travellers and Ireland: Whose Country, Whose History?* Cork University Press.

Maher, J. (1996) When the people forced change. *Irish Times,* 28 December.

Management Advisory Board (Australia) (1993) *Accountability in the Commonwealth Public Sector,* No. 11, June.

Marang-van de Mheen, P.J., Davey Smith, G., Hart, C.L. & Gunning-Schepers, L.J. (1998) Socioeconomic differentials in mortality among men within Great Britain: time trends and contributory causes. *Journal of Epidemiology and Community Health* 52 (4), Apr., 214–2188.

Marks, D. (1996) Health psychology in context. *Journal of Health Psychology* 1 (1), 7–21.

Maslow, A. (1954) *Motivation and Personality.* Harper & Row, London.

Matthews, P.A. (1996) Issues in Ireland for the Irish deaf community: an insight from a deaf person's perspective. *Teangeolas: Journal of Linguistics Institute of Ireland* 35, 12–21.

Maxwell, R.J. (1997) Quality in healthcare. *Health Service Management* 26 (2), Apr.

Mayer, G.G., Madden, M.J. & Lawrenz, E. (1990) *Patient Care Delivery Models.* Aspen, Rockville, MD.

Merton, R.K. (1969) The social nature of leadership. *American Journal of Nursing,* Dec., 2614–2618.

Milburn, K. (1996) The importance of lay theories for health promotion research and practice. *Health Promotion International* 11 (1), 41–46.

Millar, B. (1996) On goes the muzzle. *Health Service Journal,* 28 Nov., 11.

Mintzberg, H. (1996) Managing government – governing management. *Harvard Business Review,* May–June.

Mittler, P. & Mittler, H. (1994) A framework for support. In P. Mittler & H. Mittler (eds), *Innovations in Family Support for People with Learning Disabilities.* Lisieux Hall, Chorley.

Mortensen, R.A. (1994). A common language for nursing practice – a persistent dilemma: a European viewpoint. *International Council of Nurses 20th Quadrennial Congress.* ICN, Geneva.

Mulvihill, R. (1993) *Voluntary Statutory Partnership in Community Care of the Elderly.* Report 23, National Council for the Elderly, Dublin.

Murphy, K. (1996) Quality in healthcare – the patients' perspective. *8th Annual Conference, Quality Assurance in Nursing Association,* Dublin, 14 November.

Murphy, M. (1996) From prevention to 'family support' and beyond: promoting the welfare of Irish children. *Administration* 44 (2), 73–101.

Murray, S., Tapson, J., Turnbull, L., McCallum, J. & Little, A. (1994) Listening to local voices. *British Medical Journal* 308, 698–700.

Najman, J.M. (1993) Health and poverty: past, present and prospects for the future. *Social Science and Medicine* 36 (2), 157–166.

National Economic and Social Forum (1995) *Quality Delivery of Social Services.* Forum Report 6, Dublin.

National Health Service Executive (1996) *Patient Partnership: Building a Collaborative Strategy.* London.

National Nutritional Surveillance Centre (1995) *Health Status of the Irish Population, 1994.* University College Galway.

National Public Health Nursing Committee (1994) *A Service Without Walls.* IPA, Dublin.

National Rehabilitation Board (1994) *Equal Status: a Blueprint for Action.* Submission to the Commission on the Status of People with Disabilities. NRB, Dublin.

New, B. (1997) Resurrecting the notion of the 'active citizen'. *King's Fund News* 20 (2), summer, 3.

Newcastle and North Tyneside Health Authorities (1995) *Health and Healthcare in the West End of Newcastle.* Newcastle upon Tyne.

Newman, K. & Pyne, T. (1994) *Junior Doctors and Management: Preconceptions and Experience.* Middlesex University Business School.

Nolan, B. (1990) Socioeconomic differentials in Ireland. *The Economic and Social Review* 21 (2): 193–208.

Ó Cinnéide, S. (1993) Ireland and the European Welfare State. *Policy and Politics* 21 (2), 97–108.

O'Connell, P. & Rottmann, D. (1992) The Irish Welfare State in comparative perspective. In J.H. Goldthorpe & C.T. Whelan (eds), *The Development of Industrial Society in Ireland.* Oxford University Press, Oxford.

O'Donovan, O. & Casey, D. (1995) Converting patients into consumers. *Irish Journal of Sociology* 5, 43–66.

OECD (1996) *Ireland: Local Partnerships and Social Innovation.* Organisation for Economic Co-operation and Development, Paris.

Office for Health Gain (1995) *Accidental Injury in Ireland: Priorities for Prevention.*

O'Higgins, K. (1996) *Treated Drug Misuse in the Greater Dublin Area: a Review of Five Years 1990–1994.* Health Research Board, Dublin.

Oliver, M. (1983) *Social Work with Disabled People.* Macmillan, London.

Oliver, M. (1990) *The Politics of Disablement.* Macmillan, London.

O'Sullivan, T. (1994) The voluntary–statutory relationship in the health services. *Administration* 42 (1), spring.

Pavee Point & Eastern Health Board (1996) *Primary Health Care for Travellers Project.* Eastern Health Board, Dublin.

Petrie, K.J. & Weinman, J. (1997) *Perceptions of Health and Illness: Current Research and Applications.* Harwood Academic, New York.

Phillimore, P., Beattie, A. & Townsend, P. (1994) Widening in equality of health in northern England, 1981–91. *British Medical Journal* 308 (6937), 30 Apr., 1125–1128.

Pope, C. & Mays, N. (1995) Qualitative research. *British Medical Journal* 311, 42–45.

Quinn, F. (1990) Crowning the Customer. O'Brien Press, Dublin.

Quirke, B., Sinclair, S. & Kevany, J. (1994) Community participation in primary healthcare. *Administration* 42 (2), 170–182.

Rabbitte, P. (Chair) (1996) *First Report of the Ministerial Task Force on Measures to Reduce the Demand for Drugs.* Department of the Taoiseach, Dublin.

Rafferty, A. (1993) *Leading Questions: a Discussion Paper on the Issues of Nurse Leadership.* King's Fund Centre, London.

Rafferty, M. (1996) *Consultation with People with Disabilities.* Working paper, Commission on the Status of People with Disabilities, Dublin.

Reid, N.G. (1987) Nursing hours per patient: a method for monitoring and explaining staff levels. *International Journal of Nursing Studies* 24 (1), 1–14.

Review Body on Higher Remuneration in the Public Sector (1996) *Report 36 on Hospital Consultants.* Stationery Office, Dublin.

Review Group on Mental Handicap Services (1990) *Needs and Abilities: a Policy for the Intellectually Disabled.* Report of the Review Group on Mental Handicap Services, Department of Health. Stationery Office, Dublin.

Rice, F.A. (1987) The role of the nurse in health care management at policy-making level. *World of Irish Nursing,* Jan.–Feb., 5–7.

Rifkin, S. (1985) *Health Policy & Community Participation.* Croom Helm, London.

Rigge, M. (1995) Does public opinion matter? *Health Service Journal,* 7 Sept., 12–13.

Rigge, M. (1996) Sharing power. Involving patients and consumers. Health Management Guide, *Health Service Journal,* 1–3.

Robins, J. (1980) *The Lost Children: a Study of Charity Children in Ireland 1700–1900.* Institute of Public Administration, Dublin.

Ross, A. (1992) The long view of leadership. *Canadian Business,* May, 46–50.

Rossi, H., Zhijewski, L., Cavanaugh, P., Tonges, M., Brett, J. & Roy, C. (1990) *Nursing Theory: Analysis, Application, Evaluation.* Little, Brown, Boston, MA.

Sackett, D.L. *et al.* (1991) *Clinical Epidemiology: a Basic Science for Clinical Medicine.* Little, Brown, London.

Savoie, J. Donald (1995) What is wrong with the new public management? *Canadian Public Administration* 38 (1), spring.

Schumacher, E.F. (1974) *Small is Beautiful.* Sphere, London.

Scott, B.R. (1962) *An Open Systems Model,* unpublished PhD thesis, Harvard Business School.

Sermeus, W. & Delesie, L. (1992) *The Registration of a Nursing Minimum Data Set in Belgium: Six Years' Experience* (paper). School of Public Health, Leuven.

Shelley, E. (1992) *The Kilkenny Health Project: a Pilot Programme for Coronary Heart Disease Prevention in Ireland.* Project report.

Shelley, E., Daly, L., Collins, C. *et al.* (1995) Cardiovascular risk factor changes in the Kilkenny Health Project. *European Heart Journal* 16, 752–760.

Simpson, J. & Scott, T. (1997) Beyond the call of duty. *Health Service Journal*, 8 May, 2–25.

Southern Health Board (1992) *A Framework for Caring: a Review of Voluntary Organisations in the Southern Health Board Region*. Cork.

Stevenson, R. & Hegarty, M. (1994) In the picture. *Health Service Journal*, 24 Nov., 22–24.

Stogdill, R.M (1986) Personal factors associated with leadership: a survey of the literature. *Journal of Psychology* 25, 35–71.

Sutcliffe, J. & Simons, K. (1993) *Self Advocacy and Adults with Learning Difficulties*. National Institute of Adult Continuing Education, Leicester.

Sutherland, R.W. (1988) *Health Care in Canada*. The Canadian Public Health Association, Ottawa.

Task Force on the Eastern Regional Health Authority (1997) *Interim Report*, June. Dublin.

Task Force on the Travelling Community (1995) *Report of the Task Force on the Travelling Community*. Department of Equality and Law Reform, Dublin.

Thomas, S. (1996) On the right track. *Health Service Journal*, 25 Apr., 31.

Towell, D. (ed.) (1988) *An Ordinary Life in Practice*. King's Fund Publishing Office, London.

Treacy, M.M. (1988) *Setting Establishments in Nursing – a Pilot Study*. Irish Matrons' Association, Dublin.

Trinity College Dublin (1996) *Jobstown Integrated Development Project, a Community Health Response*. Department of Community Health and General Practice.

Tussing, A.D. (1985) *Irish Medical Care Resources: an Economic Analysis*. Economic and Social Research Institute, Dublin.

Van Hoesen, N. & Eriksen, L. (1990) The impact of diagnosis-related groups on patient acuity, quality of care and length of stay. *Journal of Nursing Administration* 20, 20–23.

Verheij, R.A. (1996) Explaining urban–rural variations in health: a review of the interactions between individual and environment. *Social Science and Medicine* 42 (6), 923–935.

Vincent, J. (1996) Managing risk in public services – a review of the international literature. *International Journal of Public Sector Management* 9 (2).

Walker, R. & Morgan, P. (1996) Involving doctors in management; a survey of the management development career needs of selected doctors in NHS Wales. *Journal of Management in Medicine* 10 (1), 31–52.

Wall, A. (1989) *Ethics and the Health Service Manager.* King Edward's Hospital Fund for London, London.

Wall, A. (1996) Mine, yours or theirs? Accountability in the N.H.S. *Policy & Politics* 24 (1).

Welsh Health Planning Forum (1993) *Health and Social Gain for Children: Guidance to Inform Local Strategies for Health.* WHPF, Cardiff.

WHO (1988) *Guidelines for Rapid Appraisal to Assess Community Health Needs.* Doc. WHO/SHS/NHP/88.4, Geneva.

WHO (1994) *Promoting Patients' Rights in Europe.* Geneva.

WHO/UNICEF (1978) *International Conference on Primary Healthcare.* Geneva.

Whyte, J.H. (1980) *Church and State in Modern Ireland.* Gill and Macmillan, Dublin.

Wilding, P. (1992) Social policy in the 1980s. *Social Policy and Administration* 26 (2), 107–116.

Wilkinson, R. (1996) *Unhealthy Societies: the Afflictions of Inequality.* Routledge, London.

Wilson, J. (1992) Data systems can boost nursing care. *Professional Nurse*, Feb., 325–328.

Wolf, G.A. (1986) Communication: key contribution to effectiveness – a nurse executive responds. *Journal of Nursing Administration* 16(9), 26–28.

Wolfensburger, W. (1972) *Normalisation.* National Institute on Mental Retardation, Toronto.

Wolfensburger, W. & Glen, L. (1975) *PASS 3: Programme Analysis of Service Systems,* 3rd edn. National Institute of Mental Retardation, Toronto.

Wolfensburger, W. & Thomas, S. (1981) *PASSING: Programme Analysis of Service Systems Implementing Normalisation Goals,* 2nd edn. National Institute of Mental Retardation, Toronto.

Wood, T.J., Scally G. & O'Neill, D. (1995) Management skills and knowledge required by medical directors. *Clinicians in Management* 4 (4), 2–5.

Working Group on the Implementation of the Health Strategy in relation to Persons with a Mental Handicap (1997) *Enhancing the Partnership.* Stationery Office, Dublin.

Working Party on Services for the Elderly (1988) *Report of the Working Party on Services for the Elderly.* Stationery Office, Dublin.

Workman, B. (1996) An investigation into how the health care attendants perceive their role as support workers to the qualified staff. *Journal of Advanced Nursing* 23, 612–619.

Wrigley, L. & McKevitt, D. (1995) *Professional Ethics, Government Agenda and Differential Information,* Open University Business School, Working Paper Series 95/5.

Wright, J.D. (1996) Exposing the chameleon: response to accountability and public administration. *Canadian Public Administration* 39 (2).

REFLECTIONS ON HEALTH
Commemorating Fifty Years
of the Department of Health 1947 - 1997

Edited by
Joseph Robins

279 pages   234 x 156mm   ISBN 1 872002 39 0   £16.00pbk

It is fifty years since the foundation of the Department of Health. *Reflections on Health* is a collection of critical articles reviewing the progress of Irish health and its supporting services over the intervening fifty years.

The changes that have taken place since 1947 have been dramatic. Reductions in mortality generally have given rise to increased life expectancy, 61 to 73 years for males and 62 to 79 years for females. The infant mortality rate has fallen from 68 per 1000 births in 1947 to 6 at present. There are other important considerations: the caring philosophy on which the services are now based, their availability and range, the equality of all seeking care, and the acceptance that good health is more than the absence of illness, it is a general state of well-being. While the main thrust of the health services will continue to be in the area of providing for sickness, the greatest potential for further improvement in our national health lies in the policies directed at health promotion and the prevention of ill-health. It is in this context that *Reflections on Health* reviews our national health service.

Available from bookshops, or from:-

IPA
INSTITUTE OF PUBLIC
ADMINISTRATION
Publishing Division
Vergemount Hall, Clonskeagh, Dublin 6
Tel: 01-2697011   Fax: 01-2698644
E-mail: sales@ipa.ie   Website: www.ipa.ie

Third Edition

IRISH SOCIAL SERVICES

John Curry

208 pages   216 x 138mm   ISBN 1 902448 01 4   £9.50pbk

Social services affect practically everyone in our society at some stage in their life. Two-fifths of the population depend solely or mainly on income maintenance; a third of the population is entitled to free health services; more than a quarter is engaged in full-time education; and most of the housing stock has been either provided or subsidised by the state. Just under half of all government current expenditure is devoted to the social services.

Now in its third edition, *Irish Social Services* provides an up-to-date guide to the evolution, nature and scope of the social services in Ireland – income maintenance, housing, education, health and welfare services. This book will be of particular interest to students and practitioners in the field of social administration, it will also appeal to anyone concerned with how basic social needs and problems are catered for in Ireland.

> ... a mine of information ... a vital reference work.
>
> *Evening Herald*

Publication date: Autumn 1998. Available from bookshops, or from:-

IPA

INSTITUTE OF PUBLIC ADMINISTRATION

Publishing Division
Vergemount Hall, Clonskeagh, Dublin 6
Tel: 01-2697011 Fax: 01-2698644
E-mail: sales@ipa.ie Website: www.ipa.ie